BIRTH DEFECTS

Other titles in Diseases and People

—Diseases and People—

BIRTH DEFECTS

Lisa Iannucci

 Enslow Publishers, Inc.

40 Industrial Road   PO Box 38
Box 398   Aldershot
Berkeley Heights, NJ 07922   Hants GU12 6BP
USA   UK

http://www.enslow.com

Library of Congress Cataloging-in-Publication Data

Iannucci, Lisa.
    Birth defects / Lisa Iannucci.
        p. cm. — (Diseases and people)
    Includes bibliographical references and index.
    Summary: Explains what birth defects are, efforts to treat and prevent them, and the
diagnosis of genetic and environmentally caused birth defects.
    ISBN 0-7660-1186-0
    1. Abnormalities, Human Juvenile literature. [1. Abnormalities, Human.] I. Title.
II. Series.
RG627.I26   2000
616'.043—dc21   99-16538
                                                CIP
Printed in the United States of America

10 9 8 7 6 5 4 3 2 1

To Our Readers:
All Internet addresses in this book were active and appropriate when we went to press. Any
comments or suggestions can be sent by e-mail to Comments@enslow.com or to the address
on the back cover.

Illustration Credits: Armed Forces Institute of Pathology, p. 30; Centers for
Disease Control and Prevention, p. 54; Photo provided courtesy of the Cleft Palate
Foundation, 1-800-24-CLEFT, pp. 47, 87; © Corel Corporation, p. 59 (right);
Enslow Publishers, Inc., pp. 15, 33; Photo supplied by Etymotic Research, p. 85;
Daniel Hicks, p. 59 (left); Courtesy of Pam, Rich, and Matthew McGuire, p. 75;
National Archives p. 26; National Down Syndrome Society, Helpline: 800-221-
4602, www.ndss.org, pp. 12, 43, 94, 98; Courtesy of the National Library of
Medicine, pp. 22, 69; National Pasta Association, p. 67; Images © 1995 Photo
Disc, Inc., p. 40.

Cover Illustration: © TSM/Jose L. Pelaez, Inc.

Contents

BIRTH DEFECTS

What are they? Birth defects are abnormalities that are present in an infant at birth. They include visible, structural abnormalities as well as inherited diseases.

Who gets them? Birth defects do not discriminate. All races and both sexes can be affected.

How do you get them? Birth defects are not contagious; you cannot catch them by touching someone. One or both parents can pass on a condition to their child that causes a birth defect. These birth defects are considered genetic birth defects. Other birth defects may be the result of factors outside the fetus that affect its development during pregnancy. These environmental causes include medications that the mother is taking, the medical condition of the mother, drugs, or other outside factors that alter the development of a fetus.

How are they treated? Most birth defects can be treated with medications or surgery. However, some are not treatable.

How can they be prevented? The odds of a child having a birth defect can be predicted through genetic testing, which is now available to couples considering pregnancy. It can inform parents whether they, or their fetus, are at a higher risk for having a particular disease or defect. Up-to-date vaccinations, prenatal care, and a diet that includes foods high in folic acid may help a woman prevent or reduce the number of some types of birth defects in her child. It is also important to avoid substances, such as alcohol, that can harm a developing fetus.

1

What Is Wrong with My Baby?

When an upstate New York couple was planning to have their first child, they imagined a healthy bundle of joy. Unfortunately, when their daughter was born, she was very sick. She was born with three holes in her heart and a partial narrowing of the aorta, the body's most important artery. This narrowing reduced the oxygen supply from her heart to the rest of her body, causing her to sweat, vomit, and sleep more than usual. After six and a half weeks, the baby's heart began to fail. The fragile infant and her parents were sent to a special hospital where the baby underwent emergency open-heart surgery. She survived, but would need future surgeries to help correct the defect.[1]

Neither parent thought there was a reason to be concerned about birth defects. No one in either family had a heart defect.

The mother followed her prenatal care by keeping her doctor appointments, eating right, and avoiding substances that could have harmed the fetus, such as cigarettes, drugs, and alcohol.

"We were mad at everybody, even God, but I felt like I did something wrong," said the mother. "I didn't smoke or drink and we didn't know why she had this, but I kept thinking there was something wrong with me."[2]

It is understandable that this mother was angry. After all, no one imagines having a sick baby, but it is every parent's worry. There is plenty of reason to be concerned, too, when one in every twenty-eight births is affected by at least one of the five thousand known birth defects.[3] Birth defects are conditions that are present in a child at birth. They result from changes that occur during the early stages of development of the fetus, or embryogenesis. They include heart defects, missing arms or legs, blood disorders, mental retardation, and physical disabilities.

Most birth defects are obvious at birth, but others may take a few years to develop. Birth defects can cause physical or mental impairment, and a child may die before his first birthday. According to the March of Dimes, a national organization that monitors and researches birth defects, on any given day in the United States nineteen babies die as a result of a birth defect.[4]

Julia's mother also thought she did everything right during pregnancy, but nothing could prevent what would happen to Julia. Born at nine pounds four ounces, Julia appeared to be a healthy baby. For the first six months of life, she was everything you would expect a baby to be. In the next six months, however, things changed dramatically. Julia slowly lost the ability to pull herself up, and her muscles began to weaken. After numerous tests, doctors determined that she was born with spinal muscular atrophy type II, a genetic condition that causes the muscles to deteriorate and results in paralysis. Julia died from complications of the disease when she was thirteen.[5]

Understandable Concerns

"Is our baby all right?" is usually the first question on the minds of expectant parents. In most cases, until they hold their little one, they are anxious about the health of their unborn child.

Fortunately, thanks to the advances in modern medicine, there are ways to detect or prevent some birth defects, treat others, and repair many problems that result from a birth defect. Most children can go on to live healthy lives.

Century of Advances

For millions of years, birth defects have occurred in unborn babies. Before the creation of tests that check the development of a fetus, it was impossible to determine if a child would be born with a birth defect. People born with severe retardation or deformities were often ignored, labeled social outcasts, or placed in institutions.

In this century, medical science has uncovered how some

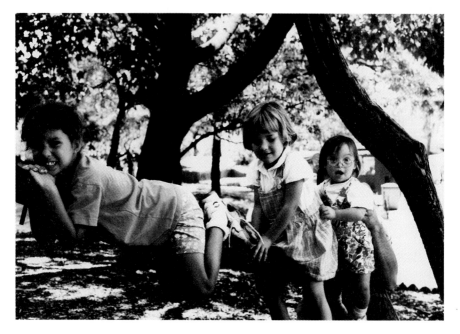

One in twenty-eight births is affected by a birth defect. In this photograph, the girl on the right has Down syndrome.

birth defects can be inherited from one or both parents. These defects are called inherited, or genetic, birth defects. Scientists have also found that birth defects can be caused by outside factors (called environmental factors), such as smoking, drugs, the expectant mother's age, the couple's health, and exposure to radiation or certain chemicals such as lead.

One example of birth defects caused by environmental factors occurred in the 1950s. Public attention was drawn to American and European mothers who were giving birth to babies with limb abnormalities. These babies were born with flipperlike arms and legs and had many other physical defects.

All these expectant mothers had taken a very powerful drug called thalidomide. This drug was prescribed by their physicians to help prevent nausea during pregnancy.

Soon after the relationship between thalidomide and birth defects was discovered, thalidomide was withdrawn from the market. Although the medication has been reintroduced into the market for the treatment of other diseases, it is not given to pregnant women or women who think they might be expecting. Other prescription drugs, including isotretinoin, which is also known by its brand name Accutane and is used to treat severe acne, have been linked to severe birth defects. Strong warnings have been issued to those who are prescribed the medication.

Scientists have also determined how various maternal diseases can cause birth defects. For example, in the 1940s, more than twenty thousand babies were born with birth defects when there was an outbreak of rubella (also known as German measles) among the pregnant mothers; over ten thousand babies died. Another condition, Rh disease, occurs when the blood of the mother and her unborn baby are not compatible. The disease once affected twenty thousand babies each year.[6] Today, Rh disease is totally preventable.

As a result of the thalidomide tragedy, the Centers for Disease Control and Prevention (CDC) in Atlanta, Georgia, began an intensive program to study the causes of birth defects. The CDC has concluded that the economic impact of birth defects is devastating: The cost for eighteen of the most severe birth defects was about $8 billion in 1992.[7]

Overcoming Birth Defects

What do actors Dudley Moore, singer Jose Feliciano, and record-setting sports stars Jim Abbott and Tom Dempsey have in common? They are all celebrities and record setters in their own rights, and they were all born with birth defects.

Moore was born with a club foot. Jose Feliciano was born blind, major-league baseball star Jim Abbott was born with half a left arm, and NFL kicker Tom Dempsey was born with a withered half-foot. Football great Boomer Esiason has a son with cystic fibrosis, and action film star Sylvester Stallone has a daughter who needed surgery as an infant to correct a heart defect. Soap opera diva Hunter Tylo (*Bold and the Beautiful*) has a baby who was born with a rare form of eye cancer and has had one eye removed.

Over the past few decades, scientists have made great strides in preventing birth defects. One of the most important discoveries revealed the link between birth defects and diet. In 1991, British researchers found that women who had previously given birth to a child with an opening along the spine, also known as a neural tube defect, had a lower chance of having other children with similar defects when they took folic acid, a B vitamin, prior to and during their pregnancy.

These studies led the U.S. Public Health Service to recommend that all women of childbearing age consume 400 micrograms of folic acid daily to reduce the risk of having a child with a neural tube defect. Many foods are now enriched with this important vitamin, including bread, rice, flour, noodles, and macaroni.[8] Folic acid can be found naturally in fruits, wheat germ, yeast breads, peanuts, and milk.

Scientists have also gained knowledge in the field of human genetics, the branch of biological science concerned with genes. Genes are units of information located on the chromosomes. Each person carries two copies of every gene, one inherited from each parent. Genes determine such information as the child's sex or hair color. Scientists have now

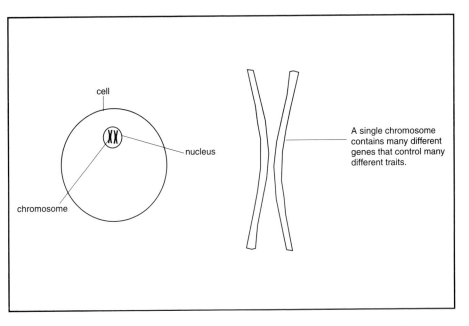

Genes are units of information on the chromosomes that determine the physical characteristics of a baby. Chromosomes are contained in the nucleus of the cell.

pinpointed specific genes that cause changes that can lead to birth defects, and they are learning how to replace the defective gene with one that works correctly.

The good news is that the rate of infant deaths due to birth defects has been cut in half since 1960. This decline results from advanced technologies, such as prenatal ultrasound, genetic testing, and specialized nurseries called neonatal intensive care units (NICUs). The decline also results from better medical management of the expectant mother, including monitoring her medical conditions, recommending good nutrition, and immunizing against infections such as rubella, as well as new treatments such as fetal surgery (operating on a fetus while it is still in the mother's womb).

Unfortunately, the causes and treatments of many birth defects are still unknown. Spina bifida, a condition in which the spine of the fetus fails to close properly during the second month of pregnancy, affects approximately one out of every two thousand babies each year in the United States. It can be mild or fatal. The scientific community believes that spina bifida may be caused by a combination of many factors. Unlike spina bifida, fetal alcohol syndrome is caused by exposure to a single drug and is completely preventable. Unfortunately it still exists. There continues to be a great deal of research and education in these areas.

Years ago, babies born with physical or mental disabilities were often institutionalized, but this practice is not as common today. You probably know people with birth defects in your town, or you may have a family member with a birth defect. Birth defects do not discriminate. Anyone, regardless of age, sex, or race, can have a child with a birth defect.

Just what is the risk that a couple will have a child born with a birth defect? What can be done to prevent birth defects? This book will help address some of these important questions and concerns.

2

The History
of Birth Defects

Throughout history, people born with visible birth defects were labeled cripples, invalids, or palsied. They were often kept away from society because of the humiliation they would endure. There was not even proper medical treatment for their condition during these times.

"Placing children with disabilities in institutions was accepted policy—indeed it was required by law in most states—until this century," says Lydia Gans in her book *Sisters, Brothers and Disability: A Family Album.* "Segregation was a humane and progressive step compared to the days when a child with a disability would be kept out of sight and treated more like an animal than a human being. Although putting children in an institution was intended to isolate them from the rest of the society, this represented a step forward by at least recognizing their humanity."[1]

Prehistoric art portrays birth defects, revealing that they existed from the earliest of times. Ancient Babylonian records show that birth defects were thought to be the sign of a displeased god. It was also commonly believed that a mother's experiences during pregnancy could shape the baby. For example, a cleft lip was thought to be caused by a mother being startled by a rabbit. A mother's encounter with a cripple was believed to cause a baby to have deformed legs.

Later, the medical community ignored these myths and tried to find reasons to explain the causes of these birth defects. In 1651, English physician William Harvey observed that some birth defects resulted from an abnormality in development of an embryo. (An embryo is the stage of growth between the time a fertilized egg is implanted in the uterus— about a week after conception—until the end of the seventh or eighth week of pregnancy.) However, further studies on animals and humans were not done until the nineteenth century.[2]

Since the mid-1800s, there have been great strides in identifying birth defects. For example, in 1866, John Langdon Down recognized certain physical traits in babies, such as slanted eyes and an enlarged tongue, that came to be known as Down syndrome. In the 1880s the findings of British ophthalmologist Warren Tay and New York neurologist Bernard Sachs helped to identify Tay-Sachs disease, a fatal, inherited disease of the central nervous system.

In 1896, Dr. Antoine Marfan examined a five-year-old patient with elongated fingers and limbs and other abnormal features of her skeleton. This condition became known as Marfan's syndrome.

The early 1900s saw more identification of birth defects, including thalassemia, an inherited disease of the blood. Thalassemia is also known as Cooley's anemia, named after the doctor who first described it in 1925. Cystic fibrosis, a fatal birth defect that causes the body to produce an abnormal amount of thick, sticky mucus and can prevent the lungs from working properly, was first identified in 1938.

The Life They Led

In the late 1800s, those living with birth defects would often work as circus entertainers. In 1811, Chang and Eng, who were born joined, became the most famous of the Siamese twins. They made a career out of traveling with the circus and lived joined together until they died at age sixty-three.[3]

Louise Simpson called herself the "Moss Haired Girl" from Australia. Louise had a condition known as albinism, in which skin lacks color pigment. However, this condition had not been identified, and Simpson made a name for herself by showing off her difference. In the early 1900s, Frances O'Conner was born without arms. She was billed the "armless wonder" and learned to use her toes and feet as others use their hands and fingers.[4] Those who were unusually small (from the condition called dwarfism) or tall (gigantism) were also featured entertainers in the circus.

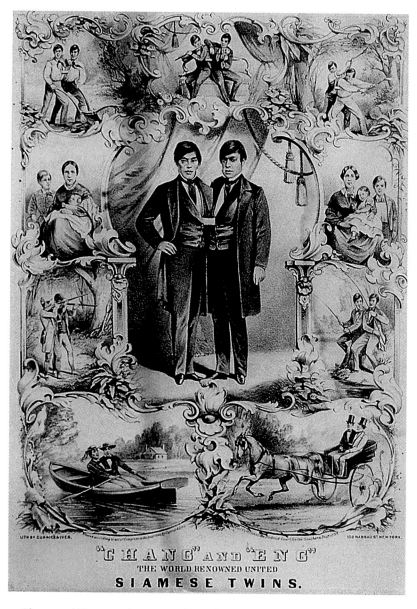

Chang and Eng were born joined together. They were the famous Siamese twins who traveled with the circus.

The most famous of these attractions was John Merrick, otherwise known as the "Elephant Man." As a child, Merrick developed large tumors over his face and body. Although fables portray Merrick's condition arising as a result of his mother's being trampled by an elephant, medical science believes otherwise. It has been theorized that Merrick had an extremely rare case of neurofibromatosis, a nervous system disorder that was first described in 1882. In 1979, scientists discovered that Proteus syndrome, an even rarer disease, seemed to fit his symptoms.[5]

German dictator Adolf Hitler was reported to have killed up to two hundred thousand disabled German citizens in the 1930s and 1940s, including many children born with birth defects.[6]

Before there were scientific advancements in the treatment of birth defects, American parents were urged to let their child die if he or she were born with severe birth defects. It was believed that these children could not go to school, learn, or play like other children, and therefore should not be allowed to suffer.

In 1982, controversy surrounded one child who was born with severe Down syndrome. The parents were told by their physician that the child would not obtain even a minimal quality of life. The parents chose to withhold the infant's feedings at the hospital and the child starved to death, although some hospital personnel attempted to interfere and save the child's life. As a result of this child's death, the Child Abuse Prevention and Treatment Act was passed to protect children born with birth defects. This law penalizes anyone for the "withholding of medically indicated treatment from disabled infants with life-threatening conditions."[7]

Environmental Role in Birth Defects

An embryo is highly vulnerable to toxic elements, called teratogens, from the third to the twelfth week of pregnancy. A teratogen is an outside substance, agent, or process that blocks the normal growth of the fetus. The type of defect depends on the type of teratogen. Some of the known teratogens are prescription drugs such as thalidomide, street drugs such as cocaine and marijuana, alcohol, diseases such as rubella, and toxic chemicals.

Events over the past century have brought attention to the environment's role in causing birth defects, including the effects of thalidomide, the aftereffects of living near a Texas toxic sludge, and effects of the chemicals of Love Canal.

Love Canal

During the 1940s and 1950s, the Hooker Chemicals and Plastics Corporation dumped toxic chemicals into an old canal in Niagara Falls, New York. Later, a community was built on the site. Unfortunately, the cement walls that sealed the chemicals were punctured. The puncture allowed the chemicals to flow into surrounding lakes, rivers, and wells, jeopardizing the health of many residents and their children. Soon, the rate of babies born with defects dramatically increased. These defects included blindness, blood disorders, and liver problems. Eventually, all of the Love Canal area was evacuated and the site was cleaned up, but all of the effects of the Love Canal waste dump are still not known.[8]

The Aftereffects of War

Although the use of chemicals during wartime has not yet been proven to cause birth defects, special registries have now been formed to track the incidence of birth defects among the children of veterans.

From 1962 to 1975, members of the United States armed forces fought in the Vietnam War. Exposed to the chemical Agent Orange while they were abroad, members of the military have noticed that there have been more incidents of spina bifida in the babies born since the war, as well as other birth defects.[9]

Twenty years later, one million service personnel served in the Persian Gulf War and were also subjected to very potent chemicals. Since their return, these heroes have complained of various health ailments and also noticed that their babies conceived since their return have had an increased incidence of chronic illnesses and birth defects, such as cancer, missing limbs, heart problems, and immune disorders.[10]

Texas Tragedy

Toxic chemicals were the cause of the massive crippling and deaths of dozens of babies in Brownsville, Texas, between 1988 and 1992. Some babies were born with spina bifida and

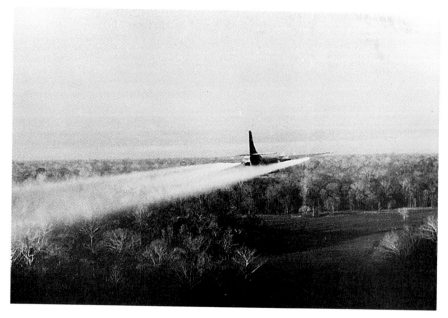

Planes sprayed the chemical Agent Orange over fields in South Vietnam during the Vietnam War. Military personnel noticed an increase in the rate of babies born with birth defects since the war.

some without full brains. Some were stillborn or died soon after being born.[11]

Directly across the border, in Montamaros, Mexico, over one hundred companies, including General Motors and Kemet Electronics, were operating factories. Mexico's lack of environmental regulations contributed to the release of toxic chemicals into the air. The families of Brownsville believed the pollution from these chemicals was killing their children. In 1997, the families won a $17-million settlement against the factories, but nothing can make up for the children who died or were crippled from this tragedy.[12]

Modern science has come a long way in recognizing, preventing, and treating birth defects, but the battle is far from over. Discovering the causes of more birth defects will help the search for prevention and treatment methods. Now that scientists have identified genes that cause birth defects, they will continue to learn how these defects can be prevented. But more research needs to be done. Not all birth defects have known causes or a means of treatment or prevention.

3
What Are Birth Defects?

A birth defect, also called a congenital defect, is a problem with the normal development of a baby during pregnancy. Some defects can be seen at birth, such as missing limbs and spina bifida. Other defects such as sickle cell anemia, Tay-Sachs disease, and some forms of muscular dystrophy do not display signs until early infancy or later. Defects can be mild and harmless, such as an extra finger. Defects can also be fatal, as with anencephaly (incompletely developed brain and skull). To understand how birth defects can happen, it is important to understand what happens when a baby is conceived.

When a baby is conceived, a mother's egg is joined by a father's sperm and a zygote is formed. The egg and the sperm each contain twenty-three chromosomes, for a total of forty-six, which are passed from the parents to the child.

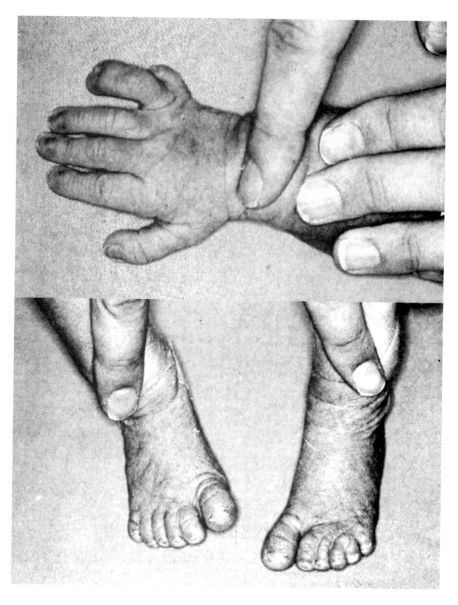

Polydactyly—having an extra finger or toe—is a mild and harmless defect.

Chromosomes are threadlike structures that are found in every cell of the body. Chromosomes have many units called genes that function as the blueprint of our bodies. Both parents contribute the genes, or pockets of information, to determine physical characteristics, including sex, hair and eye color, and height.

Cell Replication

During the twelve hours after the egg and sperm meet, the fertilized egg divides into two cells, then four cells, and so on. This process, called cell replication, continues every twelve hours for about four to five days until the fertilized egg implants itself in the uterine wall. A placenta begins to form on about the eighth day of pregnancy, when the first cells of the forming embryo join to the uterus wall. The placenta is a structure that provides the fetus with nutrients from the mother and removes waste and carbon dioxide made by the fetus. Normally, the placenta acts as a filter for many diseases and infections.

Early Pregnancy

At the end of the sixth week, the brain becomes more developed, and the arm and leg buds begin to appear. Over the next few weeks, the chest and abdomen fully form, the lungs begin to develop, and the baby's facial features form.

The embryo is called a fetus when it is eight weeks old. Virtually every organ in the fetus's body begins development during the first three months of pregnancy. At this time, the baby is very sensitive to teratogens, or toxins, that can disturb its development, including alcohol, drugs, or toxic chemicals. It is, therefore, important that the expectant mother make sure she is not exposed to these substances.

The Second Trimester

The second trimester lasts from the twelfth to the twenty-eighth week of pregnancy. At twelve weeks, the fetus has developed kidneys and eyelids. Tooth buds form and vocal cords begin to develop. The fetus begins to move, although the mother cannot feel the movements yet. The bulk of the brain growth begins to occur at the end of this trimester.

The Third Trimester

The third trimester begins at the twenty-eighth week and extends to the time of childbirth. The fetus gains most of its weight during this time. Pregnancy typically lasts anywhere from thirty-eight to forty-two weeks. By thirty-six weeks the baby is almost ready for birth, but needs to add fat to help regulate body temperature once it is born. However, if the baby is born at this time, there is an excellent chance for survival.

In most cases, the pregnancy goes well and the parents will have a healthy baby. On the other hand, three to four babies out of every hundred born will have a birth defect that occurred at some stage of pregnancy.

◯	egg	Mother's egg has 23 chromosomes.
⤹	sperm	Father's sperm has 23 chromosomes.
◯	fertilized egg (zygote)	The egg and sperm unite to form a fertilized egg with 46 chromosomes.
◖◗ ↓ ↓ ↓	zygote divides	The zygote divides many times and eventually implants itself in the wall of the mother's uterus. After development, the embryo is formed.
	9 weeks	Developing child is now called a fetus. Every organ and body system has begun development.
	12 weeks–28 weeks (second trimester)	Fetus has well developed eyes, nose, and ears. Most of the brain growth begins.
	28 weeks–40 weeks (third trimester)	The fetus gains most of its weight. At 32 weeks, the fetus is fully developed.

A fertilized egg contains chromosomes from the mother and father. In about forty weeks, a new baby will be born.

Scientists have pinpointed several genetic and environmental factors that can increase the mother's chance of having a baby with a birth defect. Chapter 4 covers genetic birth defects, and Chapter 5 introduces you to the environmental factors that can cause birth defects. In addition, the age of the mother and the number of babies being carried can affect the risk of birth defects.

Stage of Life

Recently, a woman made worldwide headlines when she announced her pregnancy. The world watched closely as she neared her due date, but not because she was a famous celebrity. It was because the mother was over sixty years old.

Fortunately, this woman delivered a healthy baby, but the risks she took were debated worldwide in the medical community. A woman's risk of having a baby with a birth defect increases as she ages. For this woman, the odds were not in her favor. Medical experts questioned her decision to risk the life of an unborn child at an age that is usually reserved for grand-mothering. Most women are not able to have children at this age because of menopause, the period ending the female reproductive phase of life, which occurs between ages forty-five and sixty.

The most common time for women to have children is during their twenties. This is considered to be the healthiest time of a woman's life to carry a child. However, many women have postponed having a child in order to focus on their careers and other goals. Over the last two decades, the number of births to women in their thirties has increased dramatically.

Many women in their thirties and forties do have healthy babies, but statistics have shown that the chances of having a baby with a birth defect are increased. For example, a twenty-five-year-old woman has a one-in-1,250 chance of having a baby with Down syndrome, whereas a thirty-five-year-old woman has greater chance, one-in-385.[1] It is believed that the cause of this increased risk is due to the decreased number of eggs a woman has as she gets older. At birth, a girl has about a million eggs in her ovaries, but as she gets older, this number decreases. The longer a woman waits to have a baby, the fewer eggs she has, and the risk increases that there may be a problem with some of them.

Teenage mothers are also at a higher risk for having a baby with a birth defect. They may sometimes be afraid and confused and may hide their pregnancies from friends and family. As a result, they may not receive adequate prenatal care. The mother's medical conditions and the baby's growth and development may not be properly monitored or treated, and potential problems may not be diagnosed. Also because teenagers may have a poor diet, the fetus can miss vital nutrients that help it grow properly.

Multiple Births

There is an increased risk of congenital defects in multiple births. A mother's body is meant to carry one baby, but sometimes a mother can carry two, three, or even more babies. (In 1998, one woman gave birth to seven babies and another gave birth to eight.) When a mother carries more than one baby, there is considerable risk of complications. Multiple babies have greater nutritional needs and put additional strains on the mother's body. The more babies a mother has, the more demands are placed on her body. As a result, the babies may be born early and can have birth defects, such as cerebral palsy.

4

Genetic Birth Defects

Just like fingerprints, no two pregnancies are alike, and for second-time mother Christine, this could not have been more true. Her first pregnancy was problem free and ended with a very easy delivery and a healthy baby girl. Her second pregnancy, however, was troublesome from day one. Christine was very sick and was hospitalized twice to stop premature labor—labor that occurs before the thirty-seventh week of pregnancy. Her doctor performed a test to check on the health of the baby and to ease Christine's fears. Unfortunately, the results of the test would do just the opposite; it would only make things worse.

Christine describes the experience as unreal, as medical personnel filed in to examine the test results. No one uttered a word or would clue Christine in. It was hours before she finally found out how seriously sick her little boy was.

Christine and her husband were told that their son had water on the brain (hydrocephaly) and spina bifida, a condition in which the spine of the fetus fails to close properly. He would need surgery to correct the problems after he was born, and might have brain damage. He might not even survive. Christine was devastated.[1]

"I wasn't able to hold him until a few days after I gave birth," says Christine. "They immediately took him away because he was having a really hard time breathing. I didn't know what was going on. They clearly stated that my son would never walk and would be mentally retarded. I felt much better when I finally had him in my arms. I was afraid that my whole world would change, but I knew I could handle anything that he had once I picked him up."[2]

Some birth defects are not diagnosed until after the baby is born. Julia, who was born healthy, stopped crawling and pulling herself up when she was six months old. She was diagnosed with a form of muscular dystrophy, a disease characterized by the progressive wasting of muscles. Eventually the muscles stop working. If the disease progresses into the involuntary muscles that control basic life functions, such as the heart muscle, the results can be fatal. Sadly, Julia died from the disease in her early teens. A few years after her first daughter was born, Julia's mother was assured by physicians that the disease was so rare it would not happen again. Unfortunately, her second daughter, Angel, has the same condition. Angel has now survived into her twenties.

"If I'm going to get worse, I can't think about it," says Angel. "I eat fruits and vegetables and take my vitamins, but I get really sick at least once a year. My doctors give me medication but whether or not I'm going to die is all up to God."[3]

It Is in the Genes

Hydrocephaly, spina bifida, and muscular dystrophy are conditions that may be caused by a change in the genes, or instructions, that direct the growth and development of the body. Genetic differences can cause minor changes, such as an extra finger or toe (polydactyly), or can cause life-threatening conditions, such as Tay-Sachs disease, which slowly affects the central nervous system. It can be the result of an altered gene or an altered gene combined with an outside factor, such as a chemical, radiation, drugs, or alcohol.

Christine's baby was born with spina bifida, or a gap in the bone that surrounds the spinal cord. The gap may be very small, in which case treatment is only rarely needed. It may, however, be large enough to allow parts of the spinal cord to stick out, in which case surgery may be needed. Spina bifida is just one of three birth defects called neural tube defects (NTDs) that affect the development of the brain and spine. Spina bifida is a birth defect that affects approximately fifteen hundred babies each year. It is believed that the condition occurs from the combination of many genes and environmental factors. The exact cause has not yet been pinpointed.[4]

Like Christine's son, children with spina bifida may have water on the brain and need treatment to remove the extra

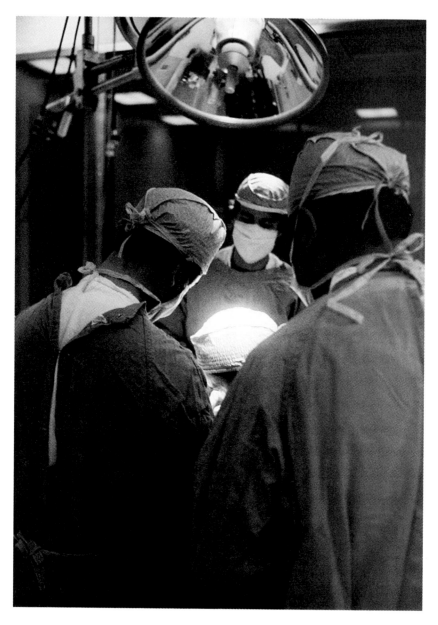

Some neural tube defects can be corrected with surgery.

fluid. This process is done through a tube, called a shunt. Without treatment, the water can build up and cause problems with brain development, and possibly mental retardation. Depending on the location of the opening in the spine, the child may suffer from bladder and kidney infections and some degree of paralysis.[5]

When the spine is exposed, serious infections can travel to the brain. Surgery is performed as soon as the baby is born to close the gap and limit the damage. Some prenatal screenings, such as ultrasound and amniocentesis, can help detect NTDs.

A Family Heritage

Genetic diseases that are considered birth defects can be inherited. A person's heritage or ethnic background can increase the risk for certain genetic diseases. For example, thalassemia and sickle cell anemia are incurable blood diseases that affect red blood cells. They are inherited diseases that can only be transmitted to the child from one or both parents who are either carriers or sufferers of the disease. Those of Mediterranean, Middle Eastern, South Asian, or African descent are at risk for thalassemia if someone in the family has passed down the specific gene. Sickle cell anemia is predominant in African-American families.

Families with northern European ancestry are at risk for cystic fibrosis—an inherited disorder of the glands that causes the glands to make very thick mucus—and phenylketonuria (PKU), a disease that prevents the body from processing food correctly. Cleft lip and palate occur more often in those of East

Asian descent and certain groups of American Indians.[6] However, a family history of a specific condition does not guarantee that the child will inherit the defect.

Chromosome Defects

Forty-six is the correct number of chromosomes to create a human being. During fertilization, however, there may be too many chromosomes. As a result, too much genetic material may be passed on to the fetus. The opposite can also occur: If there are not enough chromosomes, the embryo may lack genetic information. Both situations can lead to birth defects.

Down Syndrome

Down syndrome is one example of a chromosomal abnormality that occurs at fertilization. Also called Trisomy 21, Down syndrome is one of the most common genetic birth defects. It is the result of an extra twenty-first chromosome, either from the egg or the sperm. These extra instructions can lead to mental retardation and an increased risk for some birth defects, such as heart defects. Currently, there is no cure or prevention for Down syndrome.[7]

Children with Down syndrome have eyes that slant upward, a larger-than-normal tongue, and a small nose. They are prone to intestinal problems and hearing loss. Some of these problems are minor, others are more serious and may require surgery. Sometimes children with Down syndrome do not live very long.

In the past thirty years, the scientific community has made great strides in diagnosing and treating patients with Down syndrome. Ultrasound and alpha-fetoprotein tests are done early in pregnancy to help identify pregnancies at increased risk for Down syndrome. Fortunately, many of the problems that accompany Down syndrome can be treated. Some children with Down syndrome can attend regular school or special education classes and can live independently from their families in group homes.

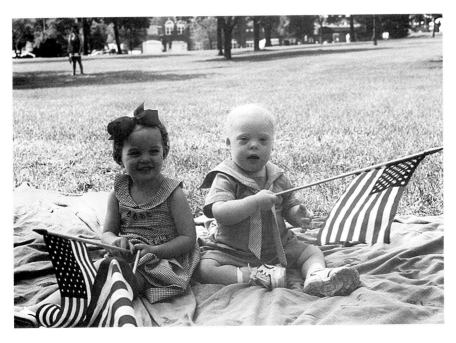

These two friends are enjoying a Fourth of July parade together. The child on the right was born with Down syndrome.

Cystic Fibrosis

Cystic fibrosis (CF) affects approximately thirty thousand children and young adults and occurs in one out of every 2,500 live births in the United States. A child must inherit an altered copy of the CF gene from each parent to have CF.[8]

Cystic fibrosis causes the body to produce an abnormal amount of thick, sticky mucus that can prevent the lungs from working properly. Children with CF need help bringing up the mucus from their lungs. Treatment may involve antibiotics, medicated vapors, or pounding on the child's back to loosen the mucus.

Other symptoms of CF include persistent coughing, wheezing, pneumonia, excessive appetite but poor weight gain, and too much salt in the child's perspiration. This excessive amount of salt is not to be confused with salty, sweaty skin that a person might have after exercising.

Genetic testing can determine if a person is a carrier of the gene that causes CF. This way, a couple knows if they are carriers and at risk for having a baby with CF. Prenatal diagnosis on the fetus includes fetal cell testing. This is done either through amniocentesis or chorionic villus sampling (CVS). After birth, a salt test can measure the amount of salt in the sweat of a child. Too much salt indicates the possibility of CF.

When CF was first identified in 1938, children with the condition usually did not live for more than six months. Today, a person with CF can survive to an average age of thirty-one years. There have also been tremendous advances in the treatment of the disease that could save more lives. In the early 1990s, scientists discovered the gene that causes CF. Scientists are now working on a method whereby a gene without mutation is incorporated into the body's cells and lessens the symptoms of CF. Gene therapy, however, is still in the future.

Over the past few years, the U.S. Food and Drug Administration has approved medications that help improve lung function in CF patients.

Sickle Cell Anemia and Tay-Sachs Disease

Sickle cell anemia is another genetic birth defect that can be passed from the parents to their child. African Americans are at an increased risk for carrying a gene that can cause the disease. When a person has sickle cell anemia, the oxygen-carrying red blood cells that are normally shaped like donuts become shaped like a sickle. They do not carry oxygen properly. The sickle-shaped red blood cells get stuck as they travel inside the small blood vessels, called capillaries, and cause the blood to stop circulating oxygen. When this happens, oxygen is not delivered to those blocked areas of the body. Individuals with sickle cell anemia develop painful aches in their arms and legs as a result. They are also at a higher risk for contracting a serious type of bacterial infection and have to be watched carefully for any signs of illness.[9]

Some Central and Eastern European (Ashkenazi) Jews carry the gene for Tay-Sachs disease, a fatal condition in which children lack an enzyme for breaking down fatty substances in the brain and nerve cells. These fatty substances destroy the brain and nerve cells, eventually causing the nervous system to stop working. Children with Tay-Sachs usually die before their fifth birthday.[10]

Prenatal tests such as amniocentesis and chorionic villus sampling can also diagnose Tay-Sachs disease, but there is no cure and no treatment.

Oral Clefts

An oral cleft occurs when either the lip or the roof of the mouth have not grown together properly in the unborn baby. A cleft palate is a split in the roof of the mouth and a cleft lip is a split through the upper lip. Research indicates that cleft lip and cleft palate result from a combination of genetic and environmental factors. Environmental factors include drugs or vitamin deficiencies that interfere with development of these structures.[11]

Babies have a one-in-700 chance of having an oral cleft and an even higher risk if another family member has been born with a cleft. Clefts can cause feeding problems, ear abnormalities, and delays in speech development. With the help of a pediatrician and plastic surgeon, the problem is usually corrected during the first three months of life. Later on, other specialists, including a psychologist, speech therapist, and dentist, may help to treat the child. Thanks to advanced surgical procedures, children with oral clefts are usually left with only a few minor scars.

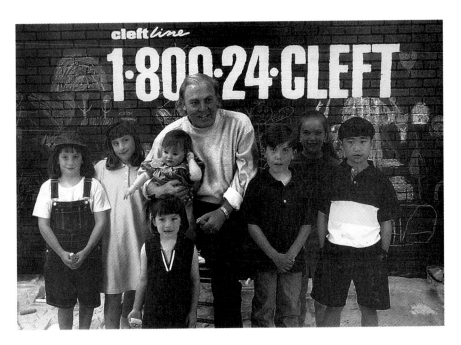

"A facial birth defect doesn't get in the way of achievement," says actor Stacy Keach, honorary chairman of the Cleft Palate Foundation. "Parents need to instill a positive sense of self-esteem in their children so they can pursue their dreams."

Heart Defects

Approximately twenty-five thousand children are born with heart defects each year.[12] Heart defects can have many causes, including genetic and environmental factors. Heart defects can happen by themselves or in combination with other birth defects. Some heart defects include coarctation (narrowing) of the aorta, and holes in the heart that may either close on their own or need surgical repair. Heart defects cannot be prevented yet, but a woman can take steps to decrease her risk of having a

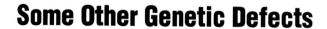

Some Other Genetic Defects

Albinism results when a child is born with little or no pigmentation of the skin. Features of this defect include ultrawhite skin and hair. The disease causes visual difficulties, lazy eye, and sensitivity to light.

Marfan's syndrome can be inherited from one parent. It is a disease of the connective tissue that results in overly tall stature and joints that bend much farther than normal. Patients can have many heart problems, including oversized heart valves, abnormal blood flow, and a weak aortic valve that can split. Sometimes sudden death occurs in adults who are unaware that they have the disease.

Immune deficiency is a problem of the immune system, which defends the body against infections and bacteria. Symptoms include infections of the ears, sinuses, and urinary tract; chronic diarrhea; weight loss; meningitis; and pneumonia. Shots of gamma globulin may help to fight infections. More severe immune deficiencies require bone marrow transplants.

Neurofibromatosis is a genetic disorder of the nervous system. Benign tumors appear under the skin and can number from one to hundreds. It is believed to be caused by a new mutation or an inherited gene. No cure is known but the effects can be treated.

Pyloric stenosis is an obstruction of the lower opening of the stomach. Surgery is required to correct this genetic defect.

baby with a heart defect. This includes testing for rubella, avoiding alcohol and drugs, and monitoring current medical conditions.

What Are the Chances?

It is possible for more than one child in a family to inherit the same defect. For example, if both parents carry the gene for phenylketonuria (PKU), an inherited disorder that affects the way the body processes food, there is a one-in-four chance that each child will have the disease.

There are inherited diseases that can be passed from both parents to a child, or just from mothers to sons. Hemophilia is an inherited bleeding disorder in which an important protein that helps the blood to clot is missing. The disease is known to pass more readily in the genes from mother to son.

5

Environmental Birth Defects

Jason is uncontrollably angry with his biological mother for causing him such difficulties in life. Jason does not have any birth defects that you can see just by looking at him, but he does suffer from severe learning disabilities, including reading problems and difficulty in memorization. He also has a tendency to be impulsive. He is not doing well in school and is frustrated at trying. He has severe psychological and behavior problems.[1]

Jason suffers from fetal alcohol effects (FAE). FAE are the result of damage from alcohol his mother drank when she was pregnant with him. The effects of his mother's alcohol use will stay with Jason for the rest of his life.[2]

Fetal alcohol syndrome (FAS) causes more damage to the fetus than FAE. Like FAE, FAS is caused by a pregnant woman's intake of alcohol during pregnancy. Affected children may have facial and heart defects and suffer from delayed growth and mental retardation. FAS can lead to stillbirths, premature births, mental retardation, and physical deformity. Over five thousand babies each year are born with FAS. Jason is one of fifty thousand babies born each year with some degree of alcohol-related damage, or FAE. Both are completely preventable. Studies have not determined exactly how much alcohol will affect the fetus, but if the mother does not drink, the risk of alcohol-related defects is eliminated.[3]

Environmental Factors

The amniotic sac cushions and protects the fetus until birth. It was once thought that nothing could penetrate the fluid or the placenta and reach the fetus, but we now know that this is not true. Toxins in the environment, such as cigarette smoke, chemicals, radiation, and viruses, can cross the placenta and reach the fetus. As a result, a baby can be born addicted to drugs or have birth defects because of its exposure to alcohol, infectious agents, or chemicals.

Diseases

During pregnancy, a woman is not immune to, or protected against, diseases such as chicken pox and rubella (German measles) unless she has had the disease or has been vaccinated. An unborn baby is vulnerable because almost everything that enters the mother's body, good or bad, is passed through to the baby via the placenta. Viruses and bacteria can cross the placenta, into the baby's bloodstream, and interfere with the normal development of the baby. The baby can contract the same disease the mother has, but the disease can sometimes harm the baby more than it harms the mother.

Chicken pox, fifth disease, group B streptococci, HIV, and hepatitis B are just some of the diseases that can pass from the mother, through the placenta, to the fetus. Whether or not the disease is going to be harmful to the fetus depends on the disease, at what point in the pregnancy the fetus contracted the disease, and the treatment available.

For example, chicken pox is a childhood illness, but it is not just for kids. If a woman has not had chicken pox by the time she becomes pregnant, she can contract the disease during pregnancy. A fetus exposed to chicken pox in the middle of pregnancy can develop pockmarks that will probably heal before birth with a minimal risk of complications. However, if the fetus is exposed to chicken pox from five to two days before delivery, the newborn can be born with a severe chicken pox infection. Without treatment, 30 percent of these newborns can die from complications. Treatment and risks all depend on when the expectant mother is exposed.[4]

Fifth disease is a common childhood illness that includes a fever, rash, joint pain, and swelling. The disease can pass to the fetus and affects the development of the fetus's red blood cells. This can lead to anemia, heart failure, and stillbirth.[5]

Rubella is a three-day form of German measles that though relatively mild for the mother can be damaging to the baby early in the pregnancy. The baby may have brain, heart,

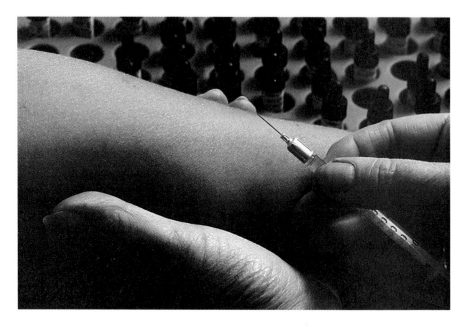

Since a mother can pass viruses and bacteria to her baby through the placenta, women should get vaccinated for diseases, such as rubella and chicken pox, before they get pregnant.

and nerve defects; mental retardation; and a delay in learning how to walk. Some may be born too small and have feeding problems.[6]

Group B streptococci are bacteria that can be transmitted from the mother to the fetus during labor and delivery and cause group B streptococci infection. The bacteria can cause breathing problems, brain damage, hearing loss, blindness, or infection in the blood in newborns. Unfortunately, many women are unaware that they harbor this bacterium in their vagina. The Centers for Disease Control and Prevention recommend a prenatal screening for strep B between thirty-five and thirty-seven weeks of pregnancy. If the mother tests positive, there are different courses of treatment, depending on the risk factors, but antibiotics are available to prevent the transmission during childbirth.[7]

Hepatitis B is a liver infection in the mother caused by the hepatitis B virus. It can pass through the placenta to the fetus, causing liver damage and premature birth. If the mother is at risk for having hepatitis B, giving her a shot of antibodies can protect the fetus.

Cytomegalovirus affects from twenty-five hundred to seventy-five hundred babies each year. The virus can cause death in newborns or numerous birth defects such as blindness and anemia. There is no treatment currently available.

Cerebral Palsy

Fetuses who are exposed to infections, such as rubella, have an increased risk of developing cerebral palsy (CP). Cerebral palsy is a group of chronic conditions that affects body movement and muscle coordination. Symptoms range from slight spastic movements of the legs to loss of muscle control, seizures, numbness, mental retardation, and blocked speech, vision, and hearing. CP can also be caused by a lack of oxygen during birth.

It is estimated that five hundred thousand children and adults have one or more symptoms of cerebral palsy, and five thousand babies are born each year with this injury to the brain. Sometimes there is damage to one or more areas of the brain during development before, during, or after birth.[8]

There are preventive measures for cerebral palsy. Routine tests for immunity to various diseases, as well as a reduction in exposure to viruses, drugs, and medications, can help prevent cerebral palsy. Prenatal care and close follow-up with the doctor is also vital.

Medical Conditions

In some cases, women have medical conditions before they become pregnant. These conditions, such as diabetes, epilepsy, and hypertension, do not prevent a woman from getting pregnant. However, if she does become pregnant, it is considered a high-risk pregnancy and must be watched closely.

A diabetic mother can have a healthy pregnancy if her blood sugar level is kept within a normal range. If not, the excess sugar can cross the placenta and cause an excess production of growth hormone in the fetus. When this happens, a fetus can grow to be very large, and this can lead to a difficult delivery. Mothers with diabetes are also at a higher risk of having a baby with a heart or spinal defect.

Medications

Sometimes the medication that controls the mother's disease causes birth defects. Antiseizure medications for epilepsy and some heart medications can cause birth defects. If it is not potentially dangerous to the mother, the physician may eliminate her medication for the duration of the pregnancy. If it will be dangerous to the mother to do so, the physician may lower or maintain the dosage and monitor the health of the baby and the mother.

The American Academy of Family Physicians reports that a pregnant woman with epilepsy may have more seizures and may fall and injure themselves or the baby. During pregnancy, a woman's body processes medications differently, which may result in a level that is too high or too low. The mother can then be at risk for seizures. Epilepsy medications can also cause bleeding, premature birth, stillbirths, and delays in development and growth.[9]

Problem Prescriptions

Thalidomide, now approved by the Food and Drug Administration for use in the United States for certain conditions, was once an experimental sedative medication that was given to pregnant women during the 1950s. The drug caused birth defects in some babies whose mothers had taken the drug. However, experimental drugs are not the only medications that may cause birth defects. Prescribed, approved medications may also increase the risk of birth defects.

Accutane was approved in 1982 to treat severe acne and is sold by prescription only. It is a vitamin A-derivative drug, but it is not a simple vitamin. Use of this potent drug increases the risk of birth defects in the children of mothers who take the medication. Accutane can cause hydrocephaly, mental retardation, small and malformed ears, and facial abnormalities.[10]

Pregnant women, or women considering becoming pregnant, should avoid Accutane or other vitamin A-related drugs. The United States government has issued strong guidelines about prescribing Accutane. Patients must be thoroughly educated about the defects this medication can cause and sign a release that states they understand the risks.

Years ago, a group of women thought to be at risk for having a miscarriage or who already had miscarriages were given a medication called diethylstilbestrol (DES). The now adolescent daughters of these women were found to have unusual cervical, uterine, and vaginal changes in their bodies.

There are occasions when a pregnant woman will get sick and need to take medication. High fevers can be very harmful to the mother and baby and must be treated. It is safe for some medications to be taken for just a day or two with the permission and supervision of a doctor.

The medical community does not know all of the effects of medications on the unborn child. Some are already recognized as dangerous and should be avoided. However, women are not always aware for the first few weeks that they are pregnant. During this time they may use medications. As a precaution, physicians recommend that all women consult their doctor before taking any medications if they suspect they might be pregnant or already know that they are.

Illegal Drugs

Illegal ("street") drugs such as cocaine, heroin, marijuana, and crack should always be avoided. All drugs taken by the pregnant mother enter her bloodstream and pass through the placenta to her unborn child. When the mother gets high on drugs, so does the baby. The amount it takes to make an adult high can do irreparable harm to a fetus. Illegal drugs can cause heart defects, missing limbs, mental retardation, brain damage, and intrauterine growth retardation, or a low birth-weight baby (five pounds eight ounces, or less). A low birthweight baby is also at a greater risk of developing breathing problems.[11]

Cigarette smoking has been linked to an increased risk of sudden infant death syndrome in babies and to an increased risk of low birthweight babies.[12]

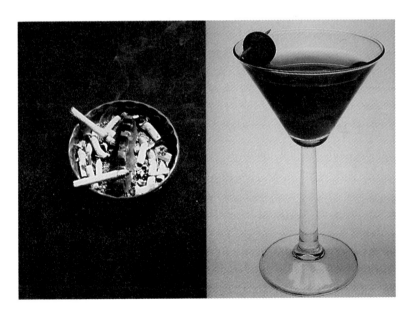

Pregnant women who smoke cigarettes and drink alcohol increase the risk of having a baby with a birth defect.

Eating Wrong for Two

Eating right throughout pregnancy is important, but it is particularly important during the first few months when the organs and brain are developing. If a mother does not eat adequately, the baby will not get the nutrients it needs. A woman who smokes, uses drugs, or drinks alcohol can also deprive the fetus of its proper nutrients. Poor nutrition can cause a baby to be born extremely small. The infant will have difficulty maintaining a normal body temperature and blood sugar level. The baby may also suffer from slow physical development.[13]

Multifactorial Causes of Defects

It is difficult to look at each birth defect or cause individually, because in many cases, the defect is the result of more than one cause. Such defects are called multifactorial. Clubfoot, in which the baby is born with a foot and ankle that are twisted out of the normal positions, is one example of a common multifactorial defect that affects one in 400 babies born in the United States each year. It is thought to be caused by a combination of genetic factors and environmental factors such as alcohol, drugs, or radiation.

6

Preventing Birth Defects

As you learned in the previous chapter, fetal alcohol effects (FAE) are caused when a pregnant woman drinks alcohol. The mother of an adopted son with FAE said,

> Anybody who is pregnant and on drugs or drinking alcohol should sit back and take a look at the child that they produced. The mother who drank or used drugs has affected someone for the rest of their lives and they are helpless because of her thoughtlessness. This child with fetal alcohol syndrome or fetal alcohol effects has to live the rest of their life with a handicap.[1]

This mother is angry. Her adopted son's FAE could have been prevented if the biological mother had not drunk alcohol while she was pregnant.[2] Similarly, if pregnant women stopped using drugs such as cocaine and heroin, the number of babies born addicted to drugs would be reduced, and the risk of birth defects related to these drugs would practically be eliminated.

Genetic Counseling

What would you do if you knew that you had a fatal disease or a condition that you could pass on to your child? It is a decision faced by many couples who want children but need to consider the risks of passing on physical or mental disabilities.

One of the century's most remarkable discoveries is the identification of genes that cause various disorders, including hemophilia, certain forms of muscular dystrophy, cystic fibrosis, sickle cell anemia, and Tay-Sachs disease. Genetic screening tests are performed on parents to determine if they are carriers of the gene that is responsible for a particular disease. The testing is done through a simple blood sample or through a sample of cells obtained from inside the mouth.

For example, cystic fibrosis is a genetic disorder that is caused by a pair of abnormal genes. Someone with cystic fibrosis has received one CF gene from each parent. These parents are called carriers. If only one parent has a gene for CF, the child will not have any symptoms of CF. If both parents have the gene for CF, together they can pass the condition on to their children.

The chance for a person to be a CF carrier depends on his or her ethnic background and is highest for white individuals with a Northern European background. However, even someone with no family history can be a carrier.

If the parents are screened, the results of genetic testing can help them to make the right choice for their situation. If they find out they are both carriers, they may decide not to have children. If the woman is already expecting, parents may choose to terminate the pregnancy, treat the child if possible (before or after birth), or simply make preparations for any complications that may arise.

Just recently, scientists have found a way to isolate some of the genes that can cause birth defects and repair or eliminate them. As a result, there is a chance that the disease can be stamped out. Unfortunately, genetic discoveries do not always guarantee a cure or effective therapy. Genetic research has allowed remarkable advances toward eliminating birth defects, but further research needs to be completed.

Anyone is eligible for genetic testing, but people with the following at-risk conditions might want to be screened before trying to have a baby: anyone who has a birth defect or has a sibling or family member with a genetic birth defect; a couple who already have a child with a genetic birth defect; or women who have had miscarriages or babies who have died as infants.

Couples concerned about their potential risk of having a child with any of the detectable conditions should discuss their options with a genetic counselor.

Obtaining Adequate Prenatal Care

Every day, an estimated 10,000 babies are born in America, 466 of which are born to mothers who receive late or no prenatal care.[3] Pregnancy is a fragile state, and there are many things that can go wrong. Prenatal care, or care during pregnancy, is vital to the good health of the mother and the

63

Advances in Gene Identification

Since the early 1980s, the scientific community has identified genetic defects for about fifty hereditary disorders, including many that do not surface until later years (Lou Gehrig's disease, Huntington's disease, and breast cancer). In the next decade, scientists hope to identify all 100,000 or more human genes through the Human Genome Project, the first step to understanding and curing genetic diseases.

Conditions for which there is genetic testing or identified genetic markers include

Down syndrome

Tay-Sachs disease

Cystic fibrosis

Sickle cell anemia

Fragile X syndrome, also called Martin-Bell syndrome

ADA deficiency, a severe and fatal inherited
    immune disorder

Acute leukemia in the fetus

Thalassemia

Marfan's syndrome

baby. It monitors the progress of the baby and keeps track of its growth, movement, and heartbeat. Based on the results of routine prenatal care, further tests can assess the health of the fetus. Otherwise, problems that can cause birth defects will not be monitored, treated, and possibly eliminated.

Ten Simple Steps to Reduce the Risks of Birth Defects

Parents should follow these ten steps:

1. Have a physical examination and have all current medical conditions checked.
2. Stop smoking.
3. Eat right.
4. Women should start taking 0.4 milligrams (400 micrograms) of folic acid every day.
5. Do not drink alcohol or use drugs.
6. Avoid toxic chemicals such as insecticides and cleaners.
7. Do not handle cat litter or eat undercooked meat, because they can lead to toxoplasmosis, an infection caused by a parasite.
8. Avoid X rays.
9. Be current on all vaccinations.
10. Schedule genetic counseling to rule out any possibility of passing on inherited disorders that could lead to birth defects.

The Food Connection

In the 1950s, scientists discovered a link between diet and neural tube defects (NTDs), such as spina bifida and anencephaly. The incidence of NTDs was higher in low-income groups in which women may have bad nutrition. In 1991, the British Medical Research Council discovered that 72 percent of women who had one pregnancy with an NTD had a lower risk for a defect in their next pregnancy when they added folic acid to their diets.

Folic acid is a B-complex vitamin that helps the body build red blood cells. It is essential for normal metabolism and helps the functioning of the nervous system, which includes the brain and spine. The need for folic acid actually doubles during pregnancy. Folate, the natural form of folic acid, can be found in animal liver and kidneys, dark green leafy vegetables, wheat germ, dried peas and beans, broccoli, asparagus, and peanuts. A woman who does not have enough folic acid in her diet is at greater risk for having a spontaneous abortion or a baby with an NTD.[4]

As a result of the British findings, the U.S. Public Health Service urged all women to include 0.4 milligrams of folic acid in their diets. Women who already had a pregnancy affected by an NTD were recommended to include a minimum of 1.0 milligram (or the equivalent of 1,000 micrograms) of folic acid in their diets. In 1995, another study reported that half of all NTDs could be prevented if a woman consumes enough folic acid *before* getting pregnant.[5] To help women meet this requirement, the U.S. Food and Drug Administration

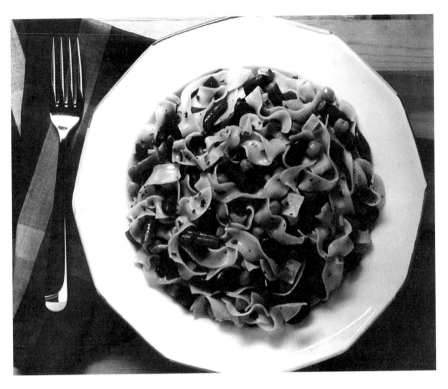

Three bean pasta is rich in folic acid, a vitamin pregnant women need to help prevent neural tube defects.

required food manufacturers to enrich grain products with folic acid.

Over the past decade the medical community has gained a positive understanding of the importance of folic acid, but the public's reaction has not been as quick. Studies by the U.S. Department of Agriculture show that many women still get only half the recommended daily amount of folic acid. In order to reap the full benefits of folic acid, women should begin taking the required dosages at least four months before getting pregnant. Since many pregnancies are unplanned, women of childbearing age should incorporate folic acid into their diets. There is much more education needed to teach the public about the benefits of this essential vitamin.

Proper Vitamin Doses

Some women are very concerned about getting the right amount of vitamins. As a result, they might take many times the recommended amount, believing that more is better. Vitamin A, which is safe in the recommended dosages, can cause birth defects among pregnant women who take more than 10,000 IUs (international units, a standard measurement of substances, including vitamins) a day. A doctor-prescribed prenatal vitamin contains only between 4,000 and 8,000 IU.[6]

Calcium supplements can also cause problems. They have been linked to harmful levels of lead, arsenic, and other heavy metals in the mother's blood, which can be transferred to the fetus.

Vaccinations

In the mid-1960s, more than twenty thousand babies were born in the United States with birth defects when their mothers contracted rubella. In 1969, a vaccination was discovered that would prevent rubella outbreaks. Women can be tested to see if they are immune to rubella. If not, a vaccination at least three to four months prior to getting pregnant will eliminate the chance of contracting the disease.[7]

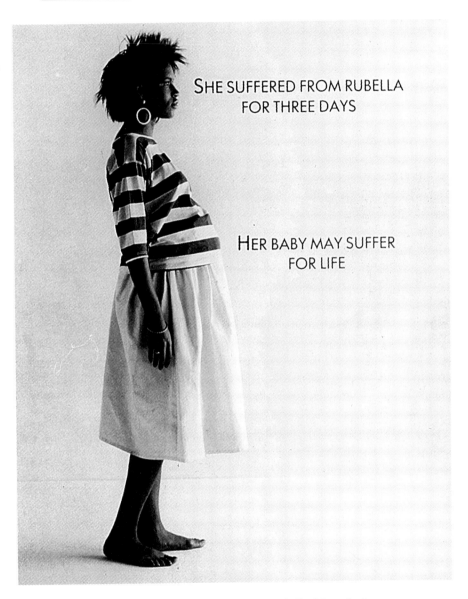

SHE SUFFERED FROM RUBELLA
FOR THREE DAYS

HER BABY MAY SUFFER
FOR LIFE

This woman did not get vaccinated against rubella. Now she is pregnant and she has caught the disease. Rubella will not have lasting effects on her, but her baby may be born deaf, blind, or both. It may also suffer heart and brain damage.

Rh disease, a condition caused when the mother's blood and the fetus's blood are not compatible, also affected 20,000 babies each year. In 1968, a treatment was created that can prevent Rh disease, and a simple blood test can tell if a woman is Rh negative. Unfortunately, mothers who need the treatment do not always get it, and at least four thousand infants each year are stillborn due to Rh disease. Rh disease can cause jaundice, brain damage, and heart failure. In severe cases, it can cause death.

Screenings

Each year, 6 percent of newborn babies die as a result of bacterial infections that the expectant mother carries, such as group B streptococcus.[8] Ten to 30 percent of pregnant women have a group B streptococci infection but are symptom free. Simple screenings can determine if the mother is carrying group B strep bacteria or other infections.

A Healthy Father

For thousands of years, modern science believed that any damage caused to a baby occurred in the woman's womb. For example, it was once thought that Down syndrome, then called mongoloidism, was caused by "uterine exhaustion," and blame was placed on the mother, not the father. It was also once believed that defective sperm are incapable of penetrating an egg. However, research has now shown that there are healthy and unhealthy sperm. Environmental factors, such as chemicals, can affect the health of the sperm, and these sperm can contribute to birth defects. Unhealthy sperm can also carry impaired genes and are capable of fertilizing an egg.[9]

This discovery has helped couples to understand that the father's health is just as important in creating a healthy baby as is the mother's health. For example, a man with a poor diet may lack vitamin C and can produce more damaged sperm than men with adequate intake of the vitamin.[10]

Method of Delivery

Sometimes how a baby is delivered, either vaginally or by cesarean section (a procedure in which the baby is surgically removed through an incision in the woman's abdomen), can decrease the risk of birth defects. For example, studies show that babies with spina bifida who are born by cesarean section have a less severe paralysis.

A Government Call to Action

The United States government has recognized the importance of preventing birth defects and in March 1998, passed the Birth Defects Prevention Act.

"Birth defects are the leading cause of infant death in America today, as well as a leading cause of childhood disability," said Dr. Jennifer L. Howse, president of the March of Dimes Birth Defects Foundation, the leading advocate of the bill. "This legislation will help us find the causes of major birth defects, devise new ways to help prevent them, and better apply what we already know."[11]

This bill assures that the National Birth Defects Prevention Study, begun in 1996, will have the money to provide the nation with a source of information on potential genetic, lifestyle, and environmental causes of birth defects. The new bill also provides funds for the expansion and improvement of existing birth defects registries and help for states that want to create them.

Currently, the CDC has three surveillance programs stationed throughout the United States and an International Clearinghouse for Birth Defects. The CDC will also provide grants to organizations for prevention programs targeted to women of childbearing age.

"The United States is one of the richest countries in the world, but the number of babies who die here before their first birthday approaches that of many developing nations. Until now, efforts to reduce the incidence of infant mortality were not receiving enough attention. This legislation will help prevent more babies from dying or having to live with disabling birth defects," says Senator Christopher Bond, a sponsor of the bill.[12]

7

Diagnosis of Birth Defects

U p until forty years ago, testing unborn babies for birth defects was not an option. Many prenatal tests were not invented or used until the mid-1900s.

Most parents want to know if their baby is healthy, and some may also wish to find out the baby's gender. Some will find out they are having more than one baby. Prenatal screens, such as an ultrasound, can be an exciting time for the parents and a big relief for those who were concerned about their baby's health. Unfortunately, this is not a happy time for all parents. Some will find out that their baby has a birth defect.

Ultrasound

Ultrasound has been used since the mid-1900s to help detect birth defects such as spina bifida and congenital heart defects. It is one of the safest forms of prenatal testing. It is painless and does not use unsafe dyes, chemicals, or radiation. Instead, it uses sound waves produced by an instrument that is waved over the mother's stomach to create an image of the fetus.[1]

Ultrasound has become an important part of prenatal care. Most expectant mothers have at least one ultrasound done during pregnancy, at approximately the sixteenth week. Ultrasound checks that the fetus is developing normally and the pregnancy is progressing without any complications.

It is an emotional experience when the expectant parents see their baby for the first time during an ultrasound on the black-and-white television screen. Little feet are kicking, hands are moving, and the baby might be sucking his thumb. The parents may ask for a printout to show family and friends or to add to the baby's scrapbook.

There are two types of ultrasound: real time and Doppler. Real time takes pictures rapidly and can detect the heartbeat, placement, and movement of the fetus. Doppler ultrasound can also be used to hear the heartbeat. Transvaginal ultrasound is a particular type of real-time ultrasound in which the ultrasound probe is inserted into the vagina and used to diagnose an early pregnancy or to assess bleeding and pain in a problem pregnancy.

The ultrasound is used to:

Verify the due date. Not all women know when they became pregnant. The ultrasound can tell them how far along the pregnancy is.

Check for more than one baby.

Evaluate the development of the fetus. Is it bigger or smaller than it should be at a particular stage of the pregnancy?

Check for possible stillbirth. An ultrasound checks for the baby's heartbeat and movement. If there is no heartbeat, the baby has died.

Check for ectopic, or misplaced, pregnancies. The fertilized egg is supposed to develop inside the uterus, but occasionally it can be found in a woman's fallopian tubes or her abdomen. This ectopic pregnancy is dangerous to the mother and the baby, and an ultrasound can detect the problem.

Determine how the baby is going to be delivered. If a baby is too large or the placenta is in the wrong place, perhaps

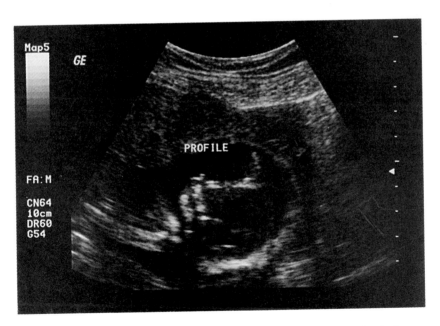

Ultrasound is an important part of prenatal care that is used to check the development of the fetus.

blocking the cervix, the baby must be delivered by cesarean section.

Ultrasounds can be done at any stage of pregnancy and are also used to detect birth defects, such as urinary tract blockages, kidney problems, missing limbs, cleft palate, and spina bifida. While it cannot diagnose Down syndrome, ultrasound has now been helpful in diagnosing certain abnormalities that are a pattern in Down syndrome, such as heart defects, gastrointestinal defects, and kidney problems. These can also be seen with other birth defects.[2]

Ultrasounds can also help to check the fetus later in pregnancy if the mother is past her due date or is having complications. The mother has a fetal biophysical profile that includes several ultrasound checks combined with a nonstress test on the baby. This test monitors the baby's movements and heartbeat while the mother lies down for a period of time.

Chorionic Villus Sampling

Chorionic villus sampling (CVS) was developed in the 1980s and is performed between the tenth and twelfth weeks of pregnancy. A catheter is inserted through the mother's vagina or a needle is inserted through the abdomen to remove a portion of the trophoblast that is part of the placenta that surrounds the embryo. The test then analyzes for chromosome disorders, such as Down syndrome or other genetic conditions, and the preliminary results are usually ready in twenty-four to forty-eight hours.

CVS can increase the risk of miscarriage and potential harm to the mother and fetus. In 1991, when tests were done between the eighth and tenth week of pregnancy, there were reports of infants born with serious limb problems and other birth defects after the procedure. CVS tests are now recommended between ten and twelve weeks of pregnancy. This change has substantially reduced the risks of miscarriage while providing vital information about possible birth defects.[3]

Maternal Serum Alpha-Fetoprotein Screening

If a mother has a higher-than-average risk of certain birth defects, such as spina bifida or Down syndrome, a relatively risk-free test called a maternal serum alpha-fetoprotein (MSAFP) screening test is performed.[4]

MSAFP measures a substance produced by the fetus: alpha-fetoprotein. Higher-than-normal levels are linked to a few major defects. Low levels are linked to a few chromosomal disorders.

If a triple-screen test is done, it means that alpha-fetoprotein, human chorionic gonadotropin (HCG), and unconjugated estriol (UE3) are tested. The triple screen has been found to be more accurate then testing only the levels of alpha-fetoprotein. The levels of these substances rise gradually during pregnancy, but if there is an abnormal reading, it may mean:

* a mistaken due date
* multiple pregnancy
* Down syndrome

* problems with the placenta, such as detachment
* low birthweight
* neural tube defects such as spina bifida or anencephaly
* abdominal defect in the muscle and skin near the belly button, called an omphalocele or gastroschisis. It is serious but can be corrected.

The MSAFP blood test is done between fourteen and twenty-two weeks of pregnancy but is best done between sixteen and eighteen weeks. The test must be done on a voluntary basis. If there are abnormal readings, follow-up will include an ultrasound or amniocentesis.

MSAFP tests can help to reassure a mother that her baby likely does not have certain birth defects, but an elevated level of MSAFP does not always mean a birth defect. There are approximately 110 women of every 1,000 who have an abnormal test result, but until further testing is done, this abnormal reading may cause the mother undue stress. If additional testing confirms a problem with the baby, parents can educate themselves on the treatment and options available to them.

Amniocentesis

Amniocentesis was used in the 1800s in the later part of pregnancy but was found to be beneficial at the early stages of pregnancy as well. Amniocentesis is now performed in some pregnant women when the fetus is from fifteen to eighteen weeks old.[5]

In amniocentesis, a sample of amniotic fluid surrounding the fetus is tested for various genetic disorders. This test is offered to women age thirty-five and older, mothers who are at risk for having a child with a birth defect, or mothers who have already had a child with a birth defect. Amniocentesis can be risky, and it increases the risk of miscarriage by almost one percent.

During the test, the physician uses ultrasound to help guide a long, thin needle into the woman's abdomen. A small amount of amniotic fluid is removed from the sac that surrounds the fetus. The fluid carries live cells from the fetus that are then taken and grown in a laboratory. Within ten to fourteen days, the cells can be analyzed for genetic abnormalities, such as Down syndrome, muscular dystrophy, and inherited disorders of body chemistry.

The results of the test are not available until late in the second trimester. In the last trimester, amniocentesis can also diagnosis uterine infections, Rh disease, and severe fetal anemia. Amniocentesis is also used as a follow-up test to the MSAFP. Alpha-fetoprotein is present in the amniotic fluid and can be measured directly in order to confirm the diagnosis of the MSAFP test.

Magnetic Resonance Imaging

Using magnetic resonance imaging (MRI), radiologists can examine the brain of a fetus to better determine if the organ is developing normally. According to a report from the Children's Hospital at the University of Pennsylvania, MRIs can detect brain abnormalities that ultrasound may not be able to pick up. No radiation is involved, and the procedure is currently done in the second and third trimesters.

Cordocentesis

Cordocentesis removes a sample of blood from the umbilical cord of the fetus to be tested for genetic abnormalities, Rh factor, and infections such as rubella and toxoplasmosis. The test is done after the seventeenth week of pregnancy and can be done until birth.[6]

What the Results Mean

A decision on what tests should be done will depend on the health and age of the mother, the expertise of the physician, what condition is being tested, and how quickly the results are needed.

A positive result in any prenatal test does not always mean there is a problem. Additional testing may be necessary to verify the positive result, or the mother may have to come back when the pregnancy is further along and the baby is more developed. Most important, however, is that the results of these tests allow parents to make informed, educated decisions about what is best for the health of their child.

What Kind of Life?

Once they find that their child will have a birth defect, parents have many options available. One choice parents have is to terminate the pregnancy, but this is not an easy decision.

Today, studies show that 80 to 90 percent of women will choose to abort when one of these prenatal tests shows a fatal abnormality such as anencephaly, in which the brain of a fetus has not finished developing and the baby will die within a short time after birth. A majority of couples will also decide to terminate the pregnancy when the baby is expected to have serious mental or physical disabilities, such as spina bifida or Down syndrome.[7]

In an article documenting a couple's decision whether or not to keep their unborn twins who were diagnosed with Down syndrome, the author wrote,

> The couple had only a few weeks to decide whether or not to terminate the pregnancy. Both had worked with [adults with Down syndrome], teaching them to shop for groceries, pay bills, and take care of their own apartments. But [the mother] also knew that some had a very hard time functioning independently, had physical disabilities, or were socially isolated. "I knew that if we had the babies I would have to reframe some hopes and dreams," says [the expectant mother]. "They might not go to college or be able to live on their own or get married." But she also felt that she could comfort herself with the thought that they would have each other.[8]

The couple chose to keep the twins.

If the parents choose not to terminate the pregnancy, they can make the necessary preparations to raise a child with a birth defect. Depending on the type of birth defect, many children can attend school and participate in the same activities that nonhandicapped children participate in. When they reach adulthood, most can live independently and have jobs and families of their own.

8
Treatment of Birth Defects

The medical community is researching birth defects to find the causes of many diseases and conditions that can harm or take the lives of thousands of babies each year. Once more causes are discovered, scientists can work on methods of preventing more types of birth defects.

In an article that documents a surgery on a fetus, Montgomery Brower wrote,

> Dr. Michael Harrison will never forget the agonizing moment he faced seven years ago in the operating room. Having opened the uterus of a Florida woman, he exposed the tiny fetus whose lethal birth defect he hoped to repair and made an incision in the unborn baby's side, Harrison saw he could go no further. Each time he attempted to pass the liver and get into the chest, the fetus's heart would stop. "We failed miserably," he said. "It broke my heart."[1]

Dr. Harrison's first failure was followed by five more in as many years, but Harrison was persistent. Blake Schultz was Harrison's first baby to benefit from revolutionary fetal surgery to repair a birth defect known as a diaphragmatic hernia. Harrison's procedure was the first ever done within the fetus itself.

"We are in a new era where fetal surgery is safe to perform in certain cases," says Medical College of Virginia plastic surgeon Dr. I. Kelman Cohen. "It is a field that will expand immensely in the next 20 years."[2]

In 1996 another fetus benefited from the advances of fetal surgery. The fetus had severe combined immune deficiency syndrome, a disorder that prevented his body from producing enough T cells. T cells are white blood cells produced by bone marrow that fight infection. Bone marrow was transplanted into the fetus, and the fighting marrow went to work where it was needed. The boy just celebrated his third birthday and is doing fine.[3]

Treatment Advances

A few years ago, both of these boys probably would have died. Today, there have been tremendous gains in the treatment of birth defects. Fetal surgery now provides hope for infants who suffer from severe birth defects such as heart damage and urinary tract blockages.

Although few birth defects can be completely corrected, the damage can be slowed, stopped, or reversed. Treatments, such as fetal surgery, can be done before the baby is born.

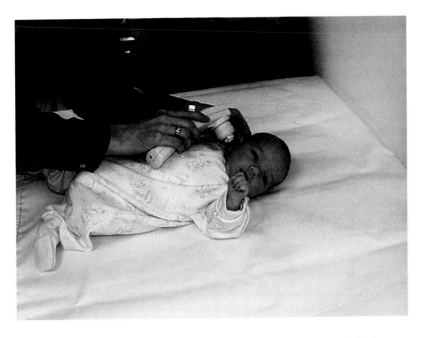

This baby is being tested with a handheld hearing tester. If the baby has a hearing difficulty, doctors can take steps to correct or improve the child's ability to hear.

Medication can be administered to reverse fetal heart failure. Transfusions can be performed to counteract Rh blood disease, and hormone therapy can be given to correct metabolic problems.

Special lifesaving equipment in intensive care nurseries and the use of a newly approved medicine, surfactant, helps low birthweight babies who otherwise might not survive. The use of magnesium sulfate by mothers who are at risk to have a child with cerebral palsy has been shown to decrease the risk of the condition.

"This intriguing finding means that use of a simple medication could significantly decrease the incidence of cerebral palsy and prevent lifelong disability and suffering for thousands of Americans," said Zach W. Hall, director of the National Institute of Neurological Disorders and Stroke (NINDS).[4]

Treatment After Birth

After birth, there are a number of treatment options to help the child survive with his disability, including surgery, rehabilitation training, medicine, therapy, and artificial limbs. Gone are the days when artificial limbs, or prosthetics, resembled Captain Hook's from *Peter Pan.* Today, nerve impulses generate movement in the artificial legs, arms, and hands to allow for beneficial opening, closing, holding, and bending. The hook has been replaced with realistic-looking fingers, toes, nails, and artificial skin. The prosthetic is made to closely resemble a human limb.

Surgical Intervention

When a baby is born with cleft lip and palate, its appearance—a slit in the lip, a deformed nose, and a hole in the roof of the mouth—can be a traumatic experience for the parents. In the past, surgery would not take place until months after the baby was born. Now, plastic surgeons operate within the first two weeks of the baby's life. Operating early allows the infant to have nearly normal functions of eating, breathing, and smiling. Children with oral clefts will undergo numerous surgeries over the years to help remove scar tissue, reshape facial features, and correct speech difficulties. Today, in most cases, the only remaining signs of the child's cleft palate and lip are the surgical scars.

Surgical procedures are also used to treat other birth defects. One form of spina bifida, meningocele, which does not involve the spinal cord and does not cause paralysis, can be corrected surgically. After surgery, children with this condition are still observed for hydrocephaly and bladder problems. Clubfoot, a common ankle and foot deformity, can also be corrected surgically. Thirty-five different kinds of heart defects can

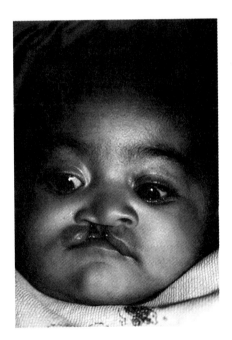 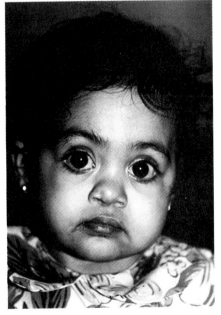

As seen on the left, Shantell was born with a complete cleft lip and palate. Doctors repaired her lip and palate with surgery.

87

now be repaired surgically, and most children who are born with heart defects can expect to live normal, productive lives.

Many defects do not have direct treatment, but there are therapies to treat the accompanying symptoms. For example, achondroplasia, or dwarfism, cannot be treated and the skeleton cannot be made normal, but the pain and pressure that accompanies the condition may be relieved through surgery. Sickle cell anemia also has no treatment, but there are therapies for reducing the severity and frequency of the pain that comes with the disease.

Transplants

Tragically, an organ such as a heart, kidney, lung, or liver can fail, and the only way to save the child's life is to remove the diseased organ and replace it with a healthy organ. Thousands of adults and children are on waiting lists for transplants, but there are just not enough donors to fill the needs of these patients.

For bone marrow transplants, the healthier the donor is, the better. Bone marrow is a soft, fatty tissue found in the bones, which creates oxygen-carrying red blood cells. Bone marrow also contains disease-fighting white blood cells, and platelets, which control clotting. Quarts of marrow are needed from donors to replace the patient's failing bone marrow. Bone marrow transplants offer children a chance for survival.

Unfortunately, it is a small chance that a bone marrow donor will match a patient. One solution to this problem is for parents to store the blood from their child's umbilical cord. The umbilical cord is the cord that attaches the fetus to the mother. This is how the baby gets its nourishment. Umbilical cord blood is rich in the cells that produce red blood cells, but the procedure is still very controversial. The blood needs to be stored and used only by family members. There is also a substantial cost for storing the blood, and the chance that it will be used is relatively slim. Scientists are still weighing the costs and benefits of this procedure.[5]

Physical Therapy

Children born with birth defects need to learn how to strengthen their muscles and how to live with their disabilities. For example, physical therapists can teach a child born with a clubfoot how to strengthen his or her foot muscles and leg muscles. They can also teach children born with spina bifida how to improve muscle ability. Physical therapists are a vital part of a team that includes a physician, a social worker, and a psychologist.

Experimental Treatments

Many treatments are still in the experimental stages and have not been approved for use in the United States. It can take decades before a drug is approved. For example, in a French study, all pregnant women diagnosed with toxoplasmosis were treated with the antibiotic spiramycin. Research shows that this medicine is effective in stopping the parasite from reaching the unborn baby. Spiramycin has not yet been approved for use in the United States.

9

What You Can Do

The first words parents may hear when their child has a birth defect are usually "we're sorry, but there is a problem," or "your baby is very sick," and they can stop a couple in their tracks. However the doctor may choose to phrase it, finding out that a child has a birth defect or disease can be devastating. The hopes and dreams of anticipating the first steps, watching a future all-star Little Leaguer, or raising a future presidential candidate are put on hold while the parents try to answer the questions, Why? and What will happen to my baby?

If a mother is informed about the defect during pregnancy, the remainder of the pregnancy can be very stressful. The mother and baby are closely monitored as the parents await the baby's birth to find out how severe the problem really is.

Once a child with special needs is born, demands on a family can be great. There may be many doctor appointments, medical tests, around-the-clock care, special diets, hospital and emergency room visits, surgeries, special programs, or therapy. The family schedule often revolves around the needs of that child.

Some siblings of a child with a birth defect are protective and proud of their brother or sister. However, siblings of that child can also feel isolated, scared, and jealous that the child with special needs is getting so much attention, and the siblings might not understand why. Older children may have to sacrifice baseball games or field trips because they interfere with the schedule of the child with special needs.

There is tremendous pressure on the parents to make sure that all of their children are given the proper amount of attention, to prevent feelings of jealousy and isolation. Marriages can suffer; the divorce rate is higher than average among parents of special needs children. There is even more burden and stress on single parent families who must handle all of these responsibilities alone.

"Taking care of our son who had been born with spina bifida was overwhelming," said Christine. "We had people coming in and out of the home and we needed help taking care of his needs, but we also had a two-and-a-half-year-old little girl who had needs too."[1]

Raising children is a big responsibility, even when a child does not have any medical concerns. Parents with children who have special medical needs can become overtired, and may be fighting their own feelings of insecurity. Many parents feel guilty that they have passed a condition or defect to their child that might have left him or her dependent on others or very sick.

"I felt terrible that I had a daughter who had a heart problem," said Maria, whose daughter was born with a severe heart defect. "I wondered what I did that caused it and why it had to happen to me and to her. I didn't want to have any more children because I was afraid that this would happen again."[2] Thankfully, Maria's second daughter, born two years later, did not have the same heart defect.

What You Can Do

"I'm a doctor who operates on children with oral clefts, but I'm also a father of two healthy unaffected children. What everyone needs to realize is that the children who suffer from birth defects didn't choose to have these conditions. You should keep in mind that interacting with these children should be done the same way you interact with any other child," says Hillel Ephros, medical director of the regional cranio-facial center at the St. Joseph's Children's Medical Center, in Paterson, New Jersey.[3]

People with disabilities face prejudice every day. These children may be judged on their looks and often ignored by nondisabled kids. As adults, it may be more difficult for them to obtain a job, and if they are hired, it is usually at less pay than a nonhandicapped person.

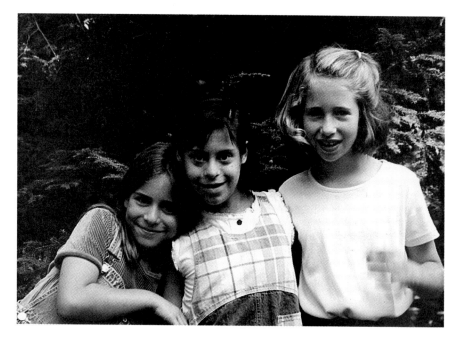

Remember that everyone likes to be treated with kindness and respect. Do not treat people with disabilities any differently from those without disabilities.

You might not be a doctor or a scientist, but there are many ways you can help eliminate or prevent birth defects, or assist those children who were born with a birth defect.

Volunteering

All organizations that dedicate their time and resources to helping children with birth defects, such as the March of Dimes, the Muscular Dystrophy Foundation, and the Cystic Fibrosis Foundation, depend on the public to carry out their missions. They need volunteers of all ages to help. Anyone can coordinate or participate in local fund-raising events, such as bowl-a-thons, walk-a-thons, and skate-a-thons. The donated money can be applied toward various needs, including research, special events for those afflicted with the condition, and tools to help the person live an easier life.

Students can also join forces with teachers for the many faculty-student competitions, such as the Cystic Fibrosis math/communications challenge, in which students complete various tests, and money is pledged toward how many answers the students get right. All this volunteering can be done in your hometown. Local chapters can help you organize any special events that you would like to plan.

If you want to focus on a specific person within your own hometown, a fund-raiser can help buy a child a wheelchair or other special equipment or start a trust fund for additional medical treatment that may be needed. Ask local physicians or hospitals for additional help to locate a family that needs help.

Hospitals also need volunteers to deliver flowers or read to sick children.

If you know a neighbor or family member who needs help caring for a disabled child, let that person know you are available. These children need a great deal of attention, and parents often do not get enough time to catch up on other responsibilities. Helping to care for the child for just a few hours a week can provide much needed rest for the parents.

Change of Attitude

Perhaps the first, most important thing that you need to do is to make sure you have the right attitude toward disabled people. You may have a friend or a sibling who was born with a birth defect. You might be embarrassed about the way they walk or talk, or you might get teased for hanging out with them. You may even feel guilty or jealous that this person needs, and receives, more attention than you do. These feelings are all valid, but you need to work them out.

If you have a brother or sister with a birth defect, you may be feeling additional pressure to help take care of him or her. You may feel as if you have to make up for any areas that the sibling is lacking in. You may also be afraid that you will get the disability, too.

If you have a friend or family member with a disability, look for a support group in your area. These support groups usually meet once a week or once a month and discuss feelings and issues regarding the disability. In a support group, you can express your opinions and concerns and discover that you are not alone. Also, make sure that your parents are aware of how you feel.

On a positive note, research has found that brothers and sisters of someone who has a disability are often mature, responsible, self-sufficient, and patient. These siblings usually grow to have a very special bond with each other.

You should eliminate certain negative words from your vocabulary. Do not call a handicapped person a "cripple" or "gimp." Remember that everyone has a weakness. Picture yourself in their position. Would you want to be called names just because you are different?

"When we went to school, we heard how we don't fit in and how we were different because we used a wheelchair," said Angel, who attended school with her sister, Julia. Both sisters were diagnosed with spinal muscular atrophy type II. "The only reason why I was different was because I like different things, not because of the wheelchair. I wish I could walk and ski, but I can't. Big deal."[4]

Treating people with respect and equality should not be limited by the color of their skin or the condition of their body. All people want to be treated fairly and respectfully. This does not change because someone is on crutches, is in a wheelchair, is blind, or has a speech difficulty.

Do Not Say "Can't"

Many disabled children participate in sports, are talented artists and writers, or play a musical instrument. They participate in programs such as the Special Olympics. They may like board games, computer games, or video games. Some disabled children just enjoy being with their families. Basically, they do not let their disability limit them.

Ten-year-old Erica Madero started life without a left arm, but that did not stop her from playing the violin. With a special prosthetic device that she uses only when she plays, Erica has performed in concerts and shows a unique passion for the instrument. She has ignored those who discouraged her from

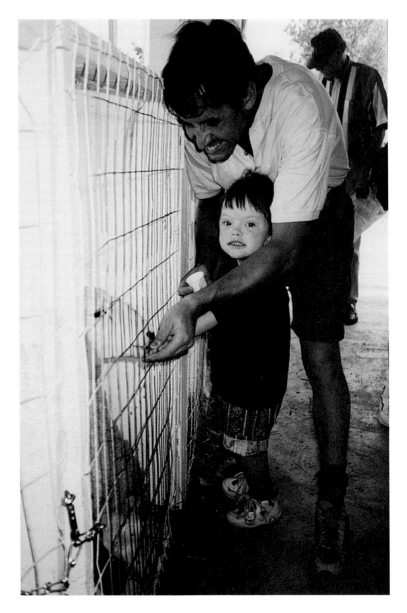

People with disabilities enjoy the same things as other people and do not let their disabilities limit them.

playing and suggested she take up an instrument easier to manipulate, like the trumpet.

"I like the way it sounds and it looked like fun," says Erica. "It was a challenge at first, because the violin is heavy and I had to get used to the weight."[5] Erica's motivation to play has inspired others with similar disabilities to learn how to play stringed instruments, and her limitations with her existing prosthesis have gotten the attention of engineers who will design a more functional artificial arm.

Eight-year-old Bryan loves to ski. He is on a soccer team and a baseball team. He is also in a weight-lifting program. Bryan was born with spina bifida and is partially paralyzed. Surprised? His mother is not. Bryan is a typical boy who enjoys sports. Thanks to special equipment and unique program opportunities, Bryan can enjoy the things that he likes to do.[6]

Communicating

If you have never talked to someone who has a disability, you might be afraid to do so. The United Cerebral Palsy Association suggests some of the following tips for talking with someone who has a handicap:

* Introduce yourself. Children with disabilities may have a hard time making friends. Introducing yourself and asking what the person likes to do may spark a common interest between the two of you.

* Sit at eye level if you are talking to a person who is in a wheelchair or on crutches.

* If the person is blind, introduce yourself once you begin speaking.

* Do not pretend to understand someone if you cannot. If it is a child, explain to the parent that you do not understand. The parent may be able to help.

* Ask questions. Do not whisper about the person or talk behind his or her back. If you have a question about someone's disability, ask. Many handicapped people would rather educate people about the disability than have people draw their own conclusions or whisper quietly.

* Before you help a disabled person, ask if he or she wants help. Many disabled persons are very capable of helping themselves. Opening a door is fine, but do not touch them or attempt to assist them without asking first.

10

The Future of Birth Defects

Hope and positive action will lead to cures," says Mandy Van Benthuysen. This energetic nineteen-year-old girl is a student government representative and manages the girls' varsity field hockey team and the boys' varsity basketball team. Mandy was homecoming princess in her freshman year in high school, and she plans to major in communications in college. Right now, she is busy serving her second year as the National Youth Chairperson for the Muscular Dystrophy Foundation.

Mandy was four years old when she was diagnosed with limb-girdle muscular dystrophy, a disease that affects the shoulders and lower trunk. She uses a wheelchair but can walk unassisted for short periods. She enjoys going out with friends to movies, school games, dances, and the beach.

"When I talk about myself to youth groups, it's to let those kids know that just because I have muscular dystrophy, it doesn't mean that I'm so different from them. As far as a cure goes, I know there will be one. I hope other people will help and contribute to make it happen."[1]

Perhaps you have seen telethons where celebrities make requests for donations to various causes. Without these funds, finding cures would be impossible. In September 1997, the Jerry Lewis Muscular Dystrophy Association Labor Day Telethon raised over $50 million in pledges and contributions to fight against neuromuscular diseases.

With these funds, MDA scientists have made dozens of important breakthroughs, including discovering the genetic causes of many neuromuscular disorders. Scientists are now working on ways to treat muscular dystrophy by altering these genes.

The March of Dimes funds scientific research to help prevent and treat the disorders. In the past, the March of Dimes has encouraged many advances, including newborn blood screening for conditions such as PKU; bone marrow transplants to treat birth defects involving the immune system; evidence linking alcohol and birth defects; ultrasonograms; treatment to prevent respiratory distress syndrome (RDS), a leading killer of premature babies; new surgical techniques to correct birth defects in the womb; and new strategies for delivering babies with spina bifida.[2]

The March of Dimes has helped to develop a new treatment using surfactant. Surfactant treatment has led to a substantial drop in deaths among babies with RDS, but 20 percent of babies do not respond to it. Scientists are continuing to look at the role of genes in RDS and trying to create different varieties of surfactant.

Down Syndrome

Today, children with Down syndrome live with their families, not in institutions; attend social functions; take music lessons; play sports; and lead normal lives. Many graduate from high school and some from college; many hold jobs and some live independently.

Babies born with Down syndrome are now being treated by a controversial vitamin therapy that has been raising hopes for these babies, but it is not an approved treatment.

Reducing Risk Factors

In 1997, scientists repaired a birth defect in a lamb by implanting the newborn with lab-grown fetal tissue. One day, this may help surgeons to repair defects in infant organs. Testing will begin on human babies within the next five years.[3]

Dr. Rochelle Hirschhorn, a professor of medicine at New York University, said, "The March of Dimes has traditionally invested in ideas that are a little ahead of their time. Someday people will look back on the era before gene therapy in the same way we now look back on the era before antibiotics and vaccines. It is now possible to think about treating a whole series of diseases with a one-shot therapy that would last a lifetime."[4]

Because of the advances in medical science, many children who would have died from certain birth defects in the past are now being kept alive. The scientific community has saved the lives of thousands of children with birth defects, but it still has more to learn.

Q & A

Q. Are birth defects contagious?

A. No. Birth defects are not contagious like a cold or flu. They are problems that occurred at some point during the pregnancy. You cannot catch a birth defect by touching a child that has a disability or by sharing toys or talking with him or her.

Q. Will a birth defect go away?

A. Some birth defects, such as a hole in the heart, can be repaired, but others cannot. For example, although some of the problems caused by Down syndrome can be repaired, the condition itself cannot be eliminated.

Q. My friends do not want to play with my sister who has Down syndrome. What should I do?

A. Explain to them that she looks different because of her condition. Instead of focusing on her looks, tell your friends about your sister; what her hobbies are and what type of music she likes. They might find that they have a lot in common with her.

Q. My brother has cerebral palsy and my parents are always taking care of him. What about me?

A. It is important to understand that children with disabilities may require special attention and help in taking care of their daily needs. Discuss your feelings with your parents and ask for some special time to spend with them.

Q. Children who do not have their sight use seeing-eye dogs to help them get around. Can I pet the dog?

A. No. The dog is there to help the child or adult and should not be distracted.

Q. Why do some children who have spina bifida wear diapers?

A. Children with spina bifida may not have bowel or bladder control. The diapers are used to prevent accidents.

Q. Someone in my school has spina bifida but he goes to regular classes. Why?

A. Spina bifida is a condition of the spine and does not affect someone's mental ability.

Q. Should I help someone in a wheelchair?

A. Ask the person first. While it is always nice to lend a helping hand, it is important to make sure the person in the wheelchair needs help. Many are capable of getting around just fine and prefer that you ask if you can help instead of just doing it.

Birth Defects Timeline

1651—English physician William Harvey observes that some birth defects result from an abnormality in the development of an embryo.

1866—John Langdon Down recognizes certain physical traits in babies, such as slanted eyes and an enlarged tongue, that came to be known as Down syndrome.

1880s—The findings of British ophthalmologist Warren Tay and New York neurologist Bernard Sachs help to identify Tay-Sachs disease, a fatal inherited disease of the central nervous system.

1896—Dr. Antoine Marfan classifies the inherited disease named Marfan's syndrome, a pattern of abnormalities that may affect the heart, blood vessels, lungs, eyes, bones, and ligaments.

1938—Cystic fibrosis, a fatal birth defect that causes the body to produce an abnormal amount of thick, sticky mucus and can prevent the lungs from working properly, is identified.

1959—Scientists determine that Down syndrome is connected to an extra twenty-first chromosome.

1990s—Scientists determine that folic acid can reduce a woman's risk of having a child with certain birth defects.

1991—Researchers identify the gene responsible for Marfan's syndrome.

1993—The National Institute of Health's first experimental dose of a gene therapy treatment for cystic fibrosis is given to an individual with the condition.

1994—Researchers identify the gene that causes achondroplasia (dwarfism).

1997—Scientists repair a birth defect in a lamb by implanting the newborn lamb with lab-grown fetal tissue.

1998—The U.S. Food and Drug Administration requires food manufacturers to enrich grain products with folic acid.

For More Information

American Cleft Palate Education Foundation
331 Salk Hall
University of Pittsburgh
Pittsburgh, PA 15261
(800) 242-5338

Association of Birth Defect Children, Inc. (ABDC)
827 Irma Avenue
Orlando, FL 32803
(800) 313-2232 or (407) 245-7035
http://www.birthdefects.org

Cleft Palate Foundation
1218 Grandview Avenue
Pittsburgh, PA 15211
(800) 242-5338

March of Dimes Birth Defects Foundation
1275 Mamaroneck Avenue
White Plains, NY 10605
(914) 428-7100
http://www.modimes.org

Sickle Cell Disease Association of America
3345 Wilshire Boulevard
Suite 1106
Los Angeles, CA 90010-1880
(213) 736-5455 or (800) 421-8453

The National Tay-Sachs and Allied Diseases Association
2001 Beacon Street
Brookline, MA 02146
(617) 277-4463

Spina Bifida Association of America
4590 MacArthur Blvd NW #250
Washington, DC, 20007-4226
(800) 621-3141 or (202) 944-3285

Chapter Notes

Chapter 1. What Is Wrong with My Baby?

1. Personal interview with Maria, December 1997.

2. Ibid.

3. The March of Dimes, *Birth Defects: A Brighter Future* (White Plains, N.Y.: March of Dimes Birth Defects Foundation, 1994), cover page.

4. March of Dimes, "On an Average Day in the United States," *The March of Dimes Infant Health Statistics*, December 1998, <http://www.modimes.org/stats/avgday.htm> (January 20, 1999).

5. Personal interview with Julia's mother, March 5, 1998.

6. John M. Bowman, "RhD Hemolytic Disease of the Newborn," *The New England Journal of Medicine*, December 10, 1998, vol. 339, no. 24, p. 1775.

7. Centers for Disease Control and Prevention, "Birth Defects, Genetic Disorders, and Developmental Disabilities Prevention and Early Intervention," March 1, 1998, <http://www.cdc.gov/nceh/programs/hp2010/oview.htm> (January 20, 1999).

8. Amy S. Kloeblen, "Women Need to Know More About Folate and Birth Defects," *The Journal of the American Dietetic Association*, January 1999, vol. 99, no. 1, p. 33.

Chapter 2. The History of Birth Defects

1. Lydia Gans, *Sisters, Brothers and Disability: A Family Album* (Minneapolis, Minn.: Fairview Press, 1997), p. v.

2. Ibid.

3. "The Personal History of Hallnson Circus Most Famous and Authentic Side Show People From Actual Historical Records," *Hallnson Circus*, n.d., <http://www.sna.com/hallnson/history.html> (January 20, 1999).

4. Ibid.

5. D. Trull, "The Elephant Man's Mistaken Identity," *Fortean Times*, #96, March 1997, <http://site034145.primehost.com/ NSGetLHP?url=%2farticles%2fo397%2felephant.htm&terms= elephant,man> (May 17, 1999).

6. Hugh Gallagher, "Slapping up Spastics: The Persistence of Social Attitudes Toward People with Disabilities," *Issues in Law and Medicine*, Spring 1995, pp. 401–414.

7. Nat Hentoff, "Getting Rid of Damaged Infants," *Village Voice*, July 1, 1997, p. 22.

8. Karen N. Peart, "Three Deadly Legacies," *Scholastic Update*, April 15, 1994, p. 6.

9. Association of Birth Defect Children, Inc., "Agent Orange," *ABDC Facts*, n.d., <http://www.birthdefects.org> (January 20, 1999).

10. Association of Birth Defect Children, Inc., "Gulf War Babies," *ABDC Facts*, n.d., <http://www.birthdefects.org > (January 20, 1999).

11. Mark Feldstein and Steve Singer, "The Border Babies: Did Toxic Waste from U.S. Factories across the Border Damage the Environment of a Texas Town?" *Time*, May 26, 1997, p. 72.

12. Ibid.

Chapter 3. What Are Birth Defects?

1. David E. Larson, *Mayo Clinic Family Health Book, Home Medical Reference* (New York: William Morrow & Co., 1996), pp. 42–46, 48, 999.

Chapter 4. Genetic Birth Defects

1. Personal interview with Christine, April 1998.

2. Ibid.

3. Personal interview with Angel, April 1998.

4. Association of Birth Defect Children, Inc., "Neural Tube Defects," *ABDC Facts*, n.d., <http://www.birthdefects.org> (January 20, 1999).

5. The Spina Bifida Program Department of General Pediatrics, *Answering Your Questions About Spina Bifida*, Children's National Medical Center, Washington, D.C., 1995.

6. L. A. Croen, G. M. Shaw, C. R. Wasserman, and M. M. Tolarova, "Racial and Ethnic Variations in the Prevalence of Orofacial Clefts," *American Journal of Medical Genetics*, August 27, 1998, pp. 42–47.

7. March of Dimes, "Down Syndrome," White Plains, N.Y.: March of Dimes Birth Defects Foundation, 1993.

8. Kerri-Lynn Lockwood, "A Family Guide to Cystic Fibrosis Genetic Testing," n.d., <http://www.phd.msu.edu/cf/fam.html> (January 20, 1999).

9. Department of Health and Human Public Health Service, *Sickle Cell Anemia: InsideMEDICINE Report*, brochure, AHCPR Publication no. 93-0564, April 1993.

10. National Tay-Sachs & Allied Diseases Association, Inc., "Tay-Sachs Disease (Classical Infantile Form)," *The NTSAD Diseases Family*, n.d., <http://www.ntsad.org/ntsad/t-sachs.htm> (January 20, 1999).

11. Harold C. Slavkin, INSIGHTS on Human Health, National Institute of Dental Research, "Meeting the Challenges of Craniofacial-Oral-Dental Birth Defects," n.d., <http://www.nidcr.nih.gov/discover/slavkin/birth_df.htm> (January 20, 1999).

12. Association of Birth Defect Children Inc., "Heart Defects," *ABDC Facts*, n.d., <www.birthdefects.org> (January 19, 1999).

Chapter 5. Environmental Birth Defects

1. Personal interview with Jason's mother, April 1998.

2. Ibid.

3. "Identification of Children with Fetal Alcohol Syndrome," *Morbidity and Mortality Weekly Report,* October 16, 1998, pp. 861–864.

4. March of Dimes, *Childhood Illnesses In Pregnancy: Chicken Pox and Fifth Disease* (White Plains, N.Y: March of Dimes Birth Defects Foundation, 1995).

5. Ibid.

6. March of Dimes, *Rubella* (White Plains, N.Y.: March of Dimes Birth Defects Foundation, 1995).

7. United Cerebral Palsy Association, "Streptococcus B Infection of the Newborn," April 18, 1998, <http://www.ucpa.org/html/research/strep.html> (January 10, 1999).

8. Judith K. Grether, "Maternal Infection and Cerebral Palsy in Infants of Normal Birth Weight," *Journal of the American Medical Association,* July 16, 1997, pp. 207–211.

9. American Academy of Family Physicians, "Epilepsy and Pregnancy—What You Should Know," *Patient Information,* July 13, 1998, <http://www.aafp.org/patientinfo/epilpreg.htm> (January 20, 1999).

10. Pauline Postotnik, "Drugs and Pregnancy," *FDA Consumer,* October 1978.

11. Rodrigo Dominguez, "Brain and Ocular Abnormalities in Infants with In-Utero Exposure to Cocaine and Other Street Drugs," *American Journal of Diseases in Children,* June 1991, vol. 145, p. 688.

12. Andrew E. Czeizel et al., "Smoking During Pregnancy and Congenital Limb Deficiency," *British Medical Journal,* June 4, 1994, vol. 308, p. 1473.

13. William Renaurd, "Prenatal Influence and the Malnourished Brain," *Nutrition Health Review,* Winter 1994, p. 7.

Chapter 6. Preventing Birth Defects

1. Personal interview with Jason's mother, April 1998.

2. Centers for Disease Control and Prevention, "Birth Defects, Genetic Disorders, and Developmental Disabilities Prevention and Early Intervention," August 21, 1997, <http://www.cdc.gov/ nceh/programs/hp2010/oview.htm> (January 20, 1999).

3. *On an Average Day in the United States, Infant Health Statistics*, March of Dimes, White Plains, N.Y., 1994.

4. L. E. Daly, P. N. Kirke, A. Molloy, D. G. Weir, and J. M. Scott, "Folate Levels and Neural Tube Defects," *The Journal of the American Medical Association*, December 6, 1995, pp. 1698–1702.

5. Ibid.

6. Roberta Larson Duyff, *The American Dietetic Association's Complete Food and Nutrition Guide* (Minneapolis, Minn.: Chronimed Publishing, 1996), p. 458.

7. *Rh Disease and Rubella*, March of Dimes, White Plains, N.Y., 1994.

8. Chris Keenan, "Prevention of Neonatal Group B Streptococcal Infection," *American Family Physician*, June 1998, p. 2602.

9. Patricia Thomas, "Reproductive Health: A Father's Role," *Harvard Health Letter*, October 1992, vol. 17, p. 5.

10. Karen F. Schmidt, "The Dark Legacy of Fatherhood," *U.S. News & World Report*, December 14, 1992, p. 94.

11. "Birth Defects Prevention Act Passed by Congress," press release by the March of Dimes, April 18, 1998.

12. Ibid.

Chapter 7. Diagnosis of Birth Defects

1. Kathy A. Fackelmann, "How Safe Is a Sonogram?" *Science News*, April 4, 1992, p. 218.

2. Robin Heise Steinhorn, "Prenatal Ultrasonography: First Do No Harm?" *The Lancet*, November 14, 1998, vol. 352, pp. 1568–1569, 1577–1581.

115

3. Leonie C. Stranc, "Chorionic Villus Sampling and Amniocentesis for Prenatal Diagnosis," *The Lancet*, March 8, 1997, vol. 349, p. 711.

4. American Family Physician, "ACOG Issues Educational Bulletin on Maternal Serum Screening," *Special Medical Reports*, March 1997, vol. 55, no. 4, <http://www.aafp.org/afp/970300ap/special3.html> (January 20, 1999).

5. James E. Haddow, Glenn E. Palomaki, George J. Knight, George C. Cunningham, Linda S. Lustig, and Patricia A. Boyd, "Reducing the Need for Amniocentesis in Women 35 Years of Age or Older with Serum Markers for Screening," *New England Journal of Medicine*, April 21, 1994, vol. 330, no. 16, pp. 1114–1118.

6. Patricia Thomas, "Fetuses Treated by Cordocentesis," *Medical World News*, June 13, 1998, pp. 95–99.

7. Mary Ellin Barrett, "The Choice I'll Never Regret," *Redbook*, August 1997, p. 84.

8. Ibid.

Chapter 8. Treatment of Birth Defects

1. Montgomery Brower, "Saving Lives Not Yet Begun," *People Weekly*, June 18, 1990, p. 38.

2. Ibid.

3. *Discover*, February 1998, p. 18.

4. National Institute of Neurological Disorders and Stroke, "Common Drug Linked to Lower Incidence of Cerebral Palsy," *Press Release*, February 8, 1995, <http://www.ninds.nih.gov/whatsnew/presswhn/1995/magnespr.htm> (January 21, 1999).

5. The Bone Marrow Foundation, "Lifeline Online," *Umbilical Cord Blood Banking*, n.d., <http://www.bonemarrow.org/umb.html> (January 10, 1999).

Chapter 9. What You Can Do

1. Personal interview with Christine, April 1998.

2. Personal interview with Maria, April 1998.

3. Personal interview with Dr. Hillel Ephros, March 1998.

4. Personal interview with Angel, April 1998.

5. Tay Pearson, "A Love of Music Knows No Barriers," *Poughkeepsie Journal,* April 2, 1998, p. 1D.

6. Personal interview with Bryan's mother, April 1998.

Chapter 10. The Future of Birth Defects

1. Muscular Dystrophy Association, "Mandy Van Benthuysen; MDA 1999 National Youth Chairperson," n.d., <http://www.mdausa.org/news/990114mandy.html> (March 22, 1999).

2. Kenneth C. Schoendorf and John L. Kiely, "Birth Weight and Age-Specific Analysis of the 1990 U.S. Infant Mortality Drop," *Archives of Pediatric and Adolescent Medicine,* February 1997, vol. 151, pp. 129–134.

3. PSL Consulting Group, Inc., *Doctor's Guide to Medical and Other News,* "Birth Defects Fixed with Fetal Surgery and Tissue Engineering," July 23, 1997, <http://www.pslgroup.com/dg/3170a.htm> (September 29, 1999).

4. New York Online Access to Health, "Genetic Testing and Gene Therapy: What They Mean To You and Your Family," *Ask NOAH About: Pregnancy,* n.d., <http://www.noah.cuny.edu/pregnancy/march_of_dimes/genetics/genetest.html> (March 23, 1999).

Glossary

amniocentesis—A procedure for obtaining amniotic fluid from a pregnant woman. A long, hollow needle is inserted through the abdominal wall into the uterus. The fluid is used to detect genetic birth defects.

birth defect—A problem with the normal development of the baby during pregnancy. Birth defects can be inherited (passed on from parent to child) or influenced by environmental factors.

cell—The basic unit of all living tissue. Within the nucleus, or center of the cell, there are the chromosomes, which determine hereditary traits.

chromosome—Found in the nucleus of a cell, chromosomes carry genes, or the individual makeup of a person.

congenital defect—Another term for birth defect. *Congenital* means "existing at birth."

DNA—Deoxyribonucleic acid. It is the carrier of genetic information.

Down syndrome—An abnormal genetic condition caused by an extra twenty-first chromosome. Also called trisomy 21.

embryo—A term for an unborn baby from conception to eight weeks of pregnancy.

enzyme—A protein that speeds up or causes chemical reactions in the body.

fetus—A term for an unborn baby after the eighth week of pregnancy.

folate—A B vitamin that is essential to the growth of an unborn baby. It should be taken daily by woman of childbearing age, especially four months prior to getting pregnant and during the first trimester of pregnancy.

folic acid—A synthetic, or man-made, version of the B vitamin folate.

gene—A unit of heredity composed of DNA and located on a chromosome. It determines characteristics such as eye color. Each person carries two copies of every gene, one inherited from each parent.

involuntary—Description of muscles that act independently or automatically, such as the heart.

mucus—A secretion of the mucous membranes, including the lining of the nose and lungs.

neonatal intensive care unit (NICU)—A special unit of a hospital that takes care of babies born prematurely or babies that need special care.

neonate—A newborn baby less than twenty-eight days old.

neural tube defects(NTDs)—Defects of the nervous system, pertaining to the spine and brain.

obstetrics—The branch of medicine dealing with pregnancy and childbirth, including the care of the mother and fetus throughout pregnancy, childbirth, and the period right after childbirth.

pediatrics—A branch of medicine concerned with the growth and care of children.

placenta—A structure through which the fetus takes in oxygen, food, and other substances and gets rid of carbon dioxide and other wastes.

premature—Describes the birth of a baby that occurs before the thirty-seventh week of pregnancy.

prenatal—Occurring before birth. The term may refer both to the care of the woman and to the growth and development of the fetus.

spina bifida—A neural tube defect that prevents the opening of the spine from closing before the baby is born.

thalidomide—A prescription drug that was given to pregnant women in the 1950s to combat nausea. It caused many birth defects, including missing arms and legs.

Further Reading

Books

Fisher, Gary, and Rhoda Cummings. *The Survival Guide for Kids with LD (Learning Disabilities)*. Minneapolis, Minn.: Free Spirit Publishing, 1991.

Gans, Lydia. *Sisters, Brothers and Disability: A Family Album*. Minneapolis, Minn.: Fairview Press, 1997.

Larson, David E., ed. *Mayo Clinic Family Health Book*. New York: William Morrow and Co., Inc., 1990.

Lutkenoff, Marlene, and Sonya G. Oppenheimer. *Spina-bilities: A Young Person's Guide to Spina Bifida*. Bethesda, Md.: Woodbine House, 1997.

Meyer, Donald Joseph, and Patricia Vadasy. *Living with a Brother or Sister with Special Needs: A Book for Siblings*. Washington: University of Washington Press, 1996.

———. *Sibshops: Workshops for Siblings of Children with Special Needs*. Baltimore, Md.: Paul H. Brookes Publishing Co., 1994.

Nilsson, Lennart. *A Child Is Born*. New York: Delacourte Press/Seymour Lawrence, 1990.

Articles

Fackelmann, Kathy A. "The Maternal Cocaine Connection: A Tiny, Unwitting Victim May Bear the Brunt of Drug Abuse." *Science News*, September 7, 1991, vol. 140, p. 152.

Goldberg, Jeff. "The Risk She Took, the Life She Saved." *Redbook*, October 1997, vol. 189, pp. 134–135.

Grant, Meg. "When the Spirit Takes Wing." *People Weekly*, May 15, 1989, vol. 31, p. 50.

Plummer, William. "Secret of a Smile." *People Weekly*, June 13, 1994, vol. 41, p. 38.

Riccitiello, Robina, and Jerry Adler. "Your Baby Has a Problem." *Newsweek*, Spring/Summer 1997, p. 46.

Schmidt, Karen F. "The Dark Legacy of Fatherhood: It's not just mothers whose habits can damage the health of their children." *U.S. News & World Report*, December 14, 1992, vol. 113, p. 94.

Internet Addresses

International Institute for Birth Defects. *Cleft.net.* 1999. <http://www.cleft.net>.

National Down Syndrome Society. *National Down Syndrome Society Website.* September 21, 1999. <http://www.ndss.org>.

The Salk Institute for Biological Studies. *The Salk Institute for Biological Studies Advances in Research on Birth Defects.* n.d. <http://www.salk.edu/advances/birthdefects/birthdefects.html>.

Shaw, Jeff. *Mountain States Genetic Network.* November 21, 2000. <http://mostgene.com>.

The Tighe Group. *Birth Defects Prevention Legislation Committee.* November 18, 1998. <http://www.birthdefectsprevention.org/index.html>.

Index

About the Author

Lisa Iannucci is a freelance health writer and has published articles in magazines, newspapers, and trade journals. She lives in the Northeast with her three children, Nicole, Travis, and Samantha. *Birth Defects* is her first book for Enslow Publishers, Inc.